STUDY MATERIAL
FOR STUDENTS OF
USUI SHIKI RYOHO
REIKI 1-2-3

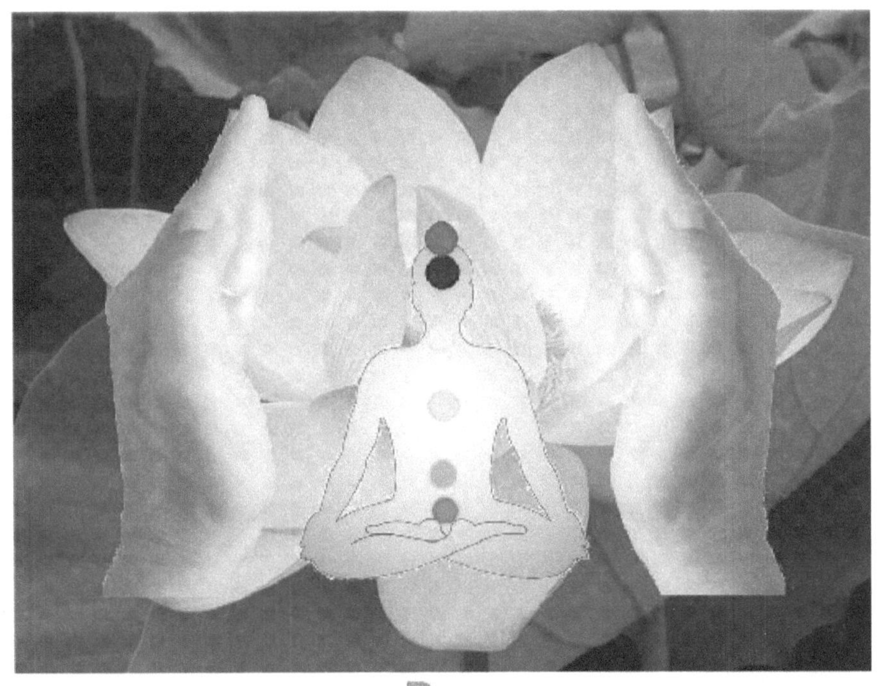

By:

DR. REKHAA KALE

STUDY MATERIAL

FOR STUDENTS OF

USUI SHIKI RYOHO

REIKI

1-2-3

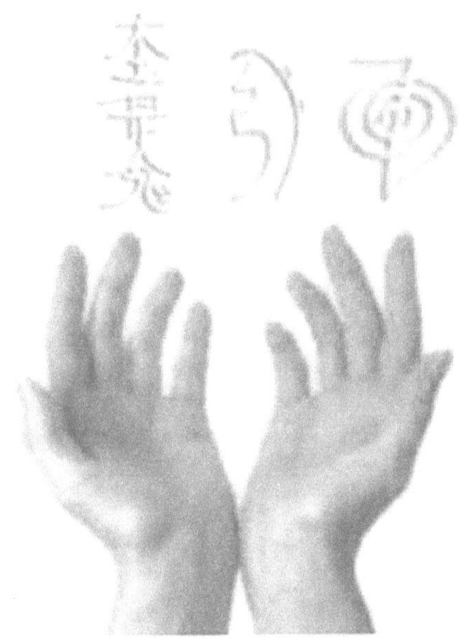

By:

DR. REKHAA KALE

PUBLISHED BY:

INTENTIONAL HEALING FOUNDATION

This is an Organization that is serving humanity since 1993. Here many methods of healing without medicines and staying physically, mentally and emotionally healthy are taught.

Reiki is the foundation of all such trainings. This is because, it creates the base of learning many ways to stay healthy and spread the message of good health.

Intentional Healing Foundation works to help society develop a healthy outlook by way of its **regular** as well as **silent social service** that all the teachers and healers working with the foundation render.

We aim to create Global Society with physical, mental, emotional, financial, family, & spiritual well-being.

We believe that a healthy mind stays in a healthy body.

All those who wish to see the surrounding healthy and happy can be a part of our foundation.

Our contact details are:

Mail: intentionalhealingfoundation@yahoo.com

Call: Founder President: Dr. Rekhaa Kale +919820044254

Social awareness work in charge Dr. Alpana Dhavale +919820461574

Training Registration in charge Ms. Sushila Doshi +919773545230

Way2Health "Teate" club in charge Ms. N. Sanghamitra +919892784933

"Energy Expressions" **ezine in charge** Ms. Neelu Sharma +61433952051

DEDICATION

Dr. Mikao Usui, many thanks to you for appearing on this planet on 15th august 1865; and giving this wonderful scientific art of healing to humanity.

Many thanks to all Master teachers trained by Dr. Usui and master teachers trained by his disciples, who took this wonderful scientific art of healing to the rest of the world. The light of knowledge spread by you masters illuminates the healing.

This book is dedicated to all the Reiki teachers and masters who directly and indirectly, physically and astrally reached me and handed over various bits of knowledge at different times. On compiling all these details, I am presenting this book for all Reiki Lovers.

Many thanks to Masters, friends, Reiki students & Reiki seekers, who helped the successful manifestation of this work.

Dear all, without your help and questions and suggestions, this perfection level in the work could never have been achieved.

5

CONTENTS:

Introduction:

Reiki is a scientific art of healing that is used to work on various types of problems. This is an art of re-establishing the lost harmony or balance in the system or even in the eco-system. This is very easy to learn and at the same time, very effective to practice. It is beyond any faith or belief.

Many teach this system of healing and as a result, there are many books written by various masters on this system. The specialty of this book is that it gives most detailed and scientific account of things taught at each level of Reiki, with the actual detailed study material of Reiki 1-2-3 levels.

As a Reiki teacher, I have been training people with Reiki and even training people to become Reiki teachers and Grand Masters since 1996, yet, let me admit that the quest into such sciences is always ongoing.

Whenever I come across something new, some new information about the methods or some new questions asked by the seekers that may be unasked questions of masses, I revise the study material used at that time, to make it more perfect; as many other teachers doing research work into Reiki.

This is how, now I am in a position to present this latest version of the study material of Reiki 1-2-3. I am sure all the Reiki practitioners and teachers are going to find it most scientific in approach, with authentic details and exhaustive material.

I would love to see the Reiki seekers benefit with this book.

Author:

Dr. Rekhaa Kale

9820044254 / 9870044254
rekhaa.kale@yahoo.com

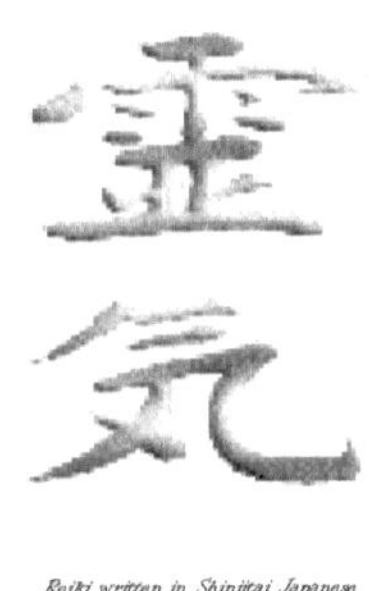

Reiki:

Reiki is a science of healing known since past century to Humanity. Since in those days, recording of teachings by writing was not common, majority of people used to remember the teachings and transmit them forward in the same way. This is the reason why, during the course of time, a number of streams were created in the Reiki teaching methods.

These streams are known as traditions of Reiki and each tradition is equally authentic as its roots are in the Reiki method that was initially taught by Dr. Mikao Usui. Let us see the various known traditions of Reiki:

Traditions of Reiki known till date:

Today many branches of Reiki are seen to exist, though there are two major traditions, respectively *Traditional Japanese Reiki* and *Western Reiki*.

Let us see these traditions in some details:

Traditional Japanese Reiki

The term *Traditional Japanese Reiki* is used to describe the specific system that formed from Usui's original teachings and teachings that did not leave Japan.

During the 1990s, Western teachers travelled to Japan in order to find this particular tradition of Reiki, though found nothing.

They therefore started to establish Reiki schools, and started to teach Reiki levels 1 and 2 to the Japanese.

Around 1993, a German Reiki Master, Frank Arjava Petter, also started to teach to the Master/Teacher level, and as a result, the Japanese started teaching their knowledge of Traditional Reiki.

Since then, several traditions of Traditional Japanese Reiki have been established, the main traditions of which are listed below.

▪ Usui Reiki Ryōhō Gakkai (臼井靈氣療法學會 in Traditional Chinese Characters, meaning "Usui Reiki Healing Method Learning Society") is the name of the society of Reiki masters founded by Mikao Usui.

Usui-Sensei, whose popular name is Mikao and whose pen name is Gyohan, came from Taniai-village, Yamagata- district, Cifu Prefecture, and had forefathers named Tsunetane Chiba who had played an active part as a military commander between the end of Heian Period and the beginning of Kamakura Period (1180-1230). His father's real name is Taneuji and his popular name is Uzaemon. His mother came and got married from the family named Kawai.

His style is assumed to have survived to the present day (assumed as no-one knows exactly how the Gakkai practises nowadays), with Ushida being the one who, upon death, substituted the presidency of the association.

This society remained secret for many years and at present, the *shihan* (master), Masaki Kondoh, is the president of the Gakkai.

Though many of their teachings still remain secret, little by little, members of this association — such as Master Hiroshi Doi — have been sharing their knowledge with the rest of the world. In spite of this, it continues to be a hermetic society, nearly impossible to access.

The power to heal is transmitted here by the method known as **Reiju**: Spiritual Blessing. In Japan, reiju is the name given to the method a teacher uses in order to communicate with individual students on an energetic level.

In the process of moving from Japan to the West, reiju changed a number of its aspects including its name. In the West its altered form is usually known as an attunement, initiation or transformation.

▪ Reidō Reiki Gakkai (靈道靈氣學會, meaning "Spiritual Occurrence and Spiritual Energy Society") is the name given to the system that derives from the masters of the Ryōhō Gakkai, and is led by Fuminori Aoki, who added to the teaching of the Gakkai, though differences in teaching are minimal.

In this system, the Koriki (meaning "the force of happiness") symbol that inspired Fuminori Aoki has been adopted.

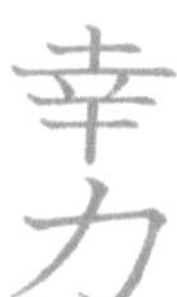

The above is the Koriki symbol used in this system. It is a very good symbol for people in depression or stress. We can hang this on wall for peace & happiness.

Reiki Healing system uses symbols to connect with specific aspects of Reiki energy, in fact to symbolize means representing some aspect in a particular way. The symbols transmitted by Usui remember his spiritual teachings. These symbols have a written or drawn and kotodama, the formula recited. They are a guide and support on the path of enlightenment that Usui pretended to teach.

The Reiki symbols are sacred, we can show and share them, but we must show respect and not use their kotodama if we are not going to activate them.

▪ **Kōmyō Reiki Kai** (光明レイキ會, meaning "Enlightened Spiritual Energy Meeting (Association)") is the name given to the system that takes the name of a school of Japanese Traditional Reiki, and was established by Hyakuten Inamoto (稲本　百天), a Reiki teacher with Western Reiki background.

It differs from other systems in that it does not originate with the Gakkai, but instead comes from the Hayashi line, through Chiyoko Yamaguchi (山口　千代子) that remained in Japan. It is based on the teachings of Dr. Chuujiro Hayashi as learned by his student Mrs. Chiyoku Yamaguchi in 1938 to 1940 (She passed away August 20, 2003 at the age of 83). But it also adds in concepts from Western Reiki and from **Gendai Reiki Ho**.

Komyo = Great light or enlightenment
Reiki = Energy of the Universe
Kai = Association or group

Komyo Reiki Kai, the system Hyakuten has created, presents Reiki as it was understood and commonly practiced in the 1930's in Japan.

This system places emphasis on spiritual unfoldment through the practice of Reiki Ryoho, aiming for "satori" or enlightenment.

Komyo Reiki is a "keep-it-simple" Reiki system and practice. The practice motto is: *"Put your hands, Surrender, and Smile"*

▪ **Jikiden Reiki** (直傳靈氣, meaning "The Direct Teaching of Spiritual Energy") is the name given to the original system that was taught by Dr. Hayashi, and was founded by Mrs. Yamaguchi and her son, Tadao Yamaguchi (山口　忠夫).

Jikiden Reiki is Usui Reiki, as this simple hand-healing method started with Mikao Usui in Japan in 1922. 'Jikiden' means directly transmitted, and in the Japanese language and culture, is a term that refers to a traditional art form, passed on carefully from teacher to student without changes.

The Japanese Reiki hand positions presented in the *Usui Reiki Ryōhō Hikkei* (臼井靈氣療法必携, *Usui Reiki Treatment Handbook*) as used and compiled by Usui are considerably more extensive than hand positions used in Western Reiki.

Mrs. Yamaguchi referred to Hayashi-Sensei's system as "Hayashi Shiki Reiki Ryoho" (Hayashi Style Reiki Healing Method), though the certificate she received is said to have had the name Hayashi Reiki Ryoho Kenkyu-kai (Research Center) on it.

While some Japanese Reiki lineages focus primarily on spiritual development, in Jikiden-Reiki the focus is strongly on healing, however, unlike western-style Reiki, apparently Jikiden does not teach formal hand positions. Mrs. Yamaguchi maintained that she was not taught any formal hand positions.

The symbols *(shirushi)*, as used in Jikiden, are slightly different to the symbols as taught by Takata-sensei.

They also have different names - which are *not* used as mantras *(jumon)*. The way in which the symbols are used and understood is somewhat different to that of Usui Shiki Ryoho. For example, what we refer to as the 'distance symbol', Jikiden classes not as a symbol, but as a *jumon*.

Western Reiki (西洋レイキ, *Seiyō reiki*) is a system that can be accredited to Hawayo Takata. The principal difference between the traditions is the use of set hand patterns for internal treatments instead of *Reiji-hō*, the intuitive skill of "knowing where to place the hands."

This style of Reiki places more emphasis on the healing of ailments, and ascension to higher levels of attunement is more formalised.

After being trained by Hayashi, Hawayo Takata went back to Hawaii, taking Reiki with her. On setting up Reiki clinics, she spread it to rest of Western world.

As a result of the Second World War, Takata decided to modify the Traditional Japanese Reiki system in order to make it more understandable and credible to the mentality of the West.

▪ **Usui Shiki Ryoho** (臼井式療法 'Usui Style Healing'): Shiki means 'style, ceremony, rite, method, system, form'; and Ryoho means, 'healing method, therapy, remedy, cure' - The method taught by the Reiki Alliance and some Independent Reiki Masters.

Usui Shiki Ryoho is the name that Usui sensei gave to his practice (it roughly translates as "Usui system of natural healing") and is close to the original eastern teachings

According to James Deacon, We can perhaps say that the REAL Original Usui Shiki Ryoho involved:
No Certificates
No Levels of training
No "Treatment Guidelines"
No Reiki Principles
No Hatsurei ho
No Joshin Kokyu ho
No Byosen Reikan ho
No Reiji ho
No Nentatsu ho
No Hand Positions
No Reiju
No Kotodama
No Symbols
No Jumon
Etc...

Rather, it simply involved an emaciated, disheveled, hungry man, sitting on the ground on the slope of a mountain his body perhaps rocking slightly to and fro his hands - radiant with the newly awakened gift of 'Reiki' - cupped instinctively around an injured toe his mind owning and breathing through the pain until the blood stopped flowing and the wound, almost miraculously, began to heal...

It is not known where the name Usui Shiki Ryoho originated. Mrs. Takata did use the name Usui Shiki Ryoho on the certificates she issued to her students.

▪ **Usui Reiki Shiki Ryōhō** (臼井靈氣式療法, commonly translated as meaning "Usui's Spiritual Energy Style of Therapy", but a more literal translation is "Usui's Spiritual Energy Style of Medical Treatment" (Ryōhō (療法) meaning *medical treatment*)) is the name given to the Western system of Reiki, and is a system that has tried to stay near enough the same as the original practises of Hawayo Takata.

It is taught today by, for instance, the Reiki Alliance, led by Phyllis Lei Furumoto, Takata's granddaughter.

In this system, as with most Western systems of Reiki, there are three levels, respectively called the First Degree, Second Degree, & Master / Teacher Degree, using Takata's version of four original symbols passed to her by Hayashi.

Usui Reiki Shiki Ryōhō is also the norm requested qualification (along with Reiki lineage) when seeking insurance to practice Reiki on the general public in the United Kingdom.

▪ **Usui/Tibetan Reiki** is the name given to the system that was developed by Arthur Robertson and later popularized by William Lee Rand and Diane Stein.

This system is derived from Usui Reiki as taught by Takata and includes techniques from the Usui Reiki Ryōhō Gakkai, such as *Byōsen-hō* (病専法, *Scanning Method*), *Gyōshi-hō* (凝視法, *Healing Eyes Method*), and *Kenyoku-hō* (件抑制法, *Dry Bathing Method*).

There have been a few additions to this system in comparison with Usui Shiki Ryōhō by Rand, such as a modified attunement method that incorporates the Violet Breath, the use of the Tibetan Master and kundalini fire symbols along with the four traditional Usui symbols, the hui yin position (located in the perineum), and also the microcosmic orbit.

Along with introducing the above, Usui/Tibetan Reiki can sometimes incorporate psychic surgery. Unlike Usui Reiki Shiki Ryōhō, it has four levels, commonly called First Degree, Second Degree, Advanced Reiki Training (commonly *3A* or *ART*), and Master/Teacher (commonly *3B*).

▪ **Gendai Reiki Hō** (現代靈氣法, meaning "Modern Spiritual Energy Method") is a system that incorporates elements of both Japanese and Western Reiki, and was established by Hiroshi Doi. Doi was first trained in Western Reiki by Mieko Mitsui, a Master of the "Radiance Technique." In 1993, he was granted membership to Usui Reiki Ryōhō Gakkai.

Gendai means modern, **Reiki** is the healing energy & **ho** means method. This is relatively a new method that is just a decade or so old. It tries to simplify the teachings of Reiki as much as possible. It has the following motto:

Ayashiku-nai   = Nothing sinister
Okashiku-nai   = Nothing strange
Muzukashiku-nai = Nothing difficult

• **Healing Teate Kagakuteki** (Healing Teate Kagakuteki) means scientific presentation of Usui shiki ryoho Touch healing method. This system presents the original teachings of Sensai Dr. Mikao Usui in the most original form while interpreting everything in the most scientific manner so that every logically thinking person understands them without having to believe in it.

Over a period of time, there are many distortions in the original teachings of Dr. Usui. Also, many blind faiths and ideas that limit the actual spirit of Reiki are added to this wonderful system over past 90 years of the journey of **Usui Shiki Ryoho Reiki.** Reiki therefore is known in different ways and school names.

It was the astral blessings and teachings of Dr. Usui that has lead the foundation of this school of Reiki.

Everything stated here has come directly from Dr. Usui through astral communication to various Reiki grandmasters and teachers. So again like his system that was known as Ronin, or leaderless method, even this system is leaderless as it has come from teachings of Sensai Usui received by many different sources at different times.

Probably this is the only school of Reiki that gives training into Basic anatomy and basic counseling techniques along with regular Reiju and Training into Touch & distance healing methods, and explains all the 5 pillars of Reiki in absolute details. Here no blind faith or assumption is entertained.

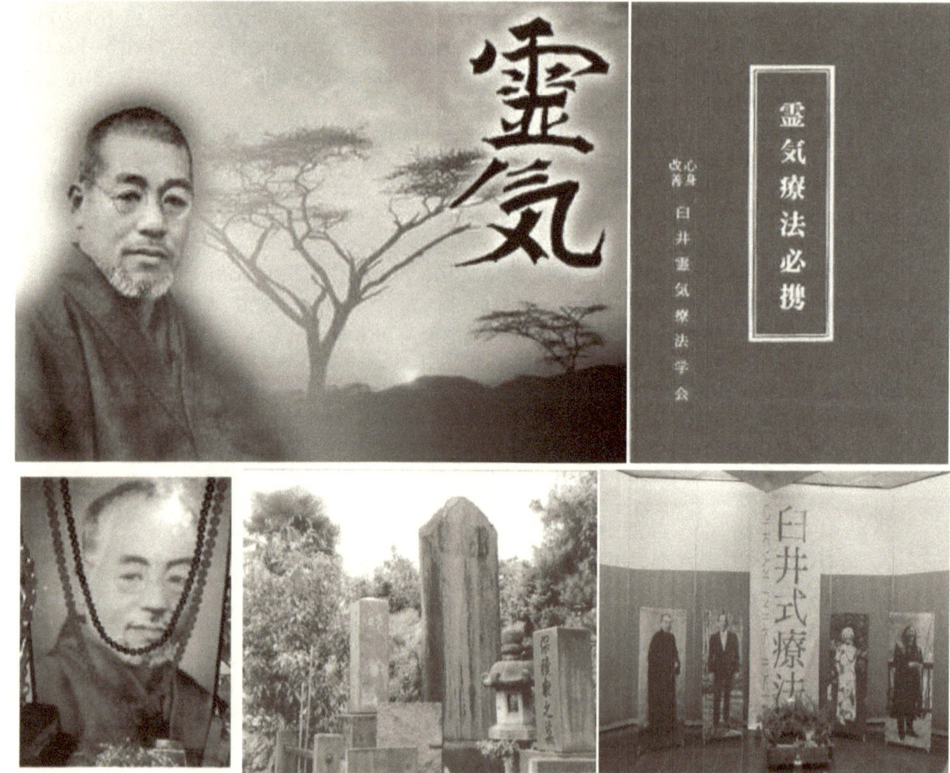

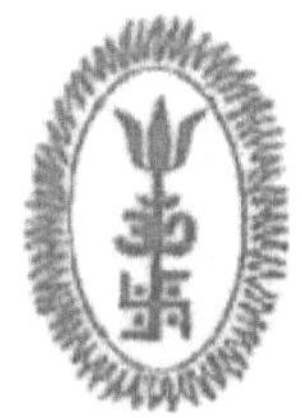

INTENTIONAL HEALING FOUNDATION

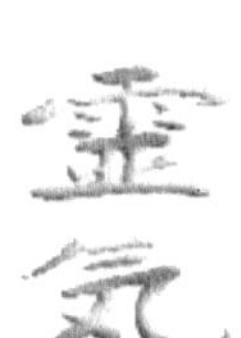
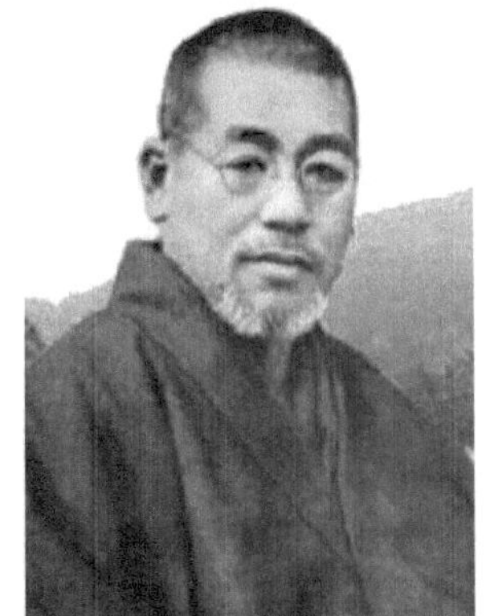
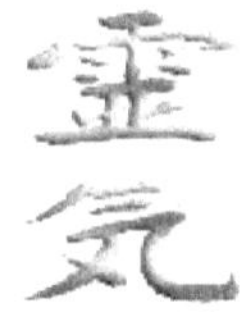

Reiki 1

STUDY MATERIAL

BY

DR. REKHAA KALE
9820044254 / 9870044254
rekhaa.kale@yahoo.com

ABOUT REIKI

Reiki is an ancient Japanese science of healing. It involves the use of REI means universal light & KI means life force energy governing all functions in universe. This helps you heal all kinds of problem by touch or thought.

This is just a complimentary aid to medicine that one can use with REJU i.e. attunement or initiation. Without initiation one cannot use it effectively. Those who try to practice this just by reading a book may get only a part of the healing effect that will be initiated with their own energy, not the universal life force.

Reiki has 10 levels. Out of this, Reiki healing is taught in 4 levels. After this, there are 4 levels of Reiki teacher, 1 level of Reiki Grand Master and 1 level of Reiki Great Grand master.

This literature of Reiki 1 will give you the basic idea of Reiki and as you get attuned, you can heal yourself as well as others by touch.

You can even heal some objects and things and places by touch if you try that too.

We have heard of some spiritually developed people doing such things earlier, but I am sure you must never have believed those stories to be true.

Now, as you get attuned into Reiki, you will realise that even you can do this. Naturally you will know that this works.

In Reiki 2, you will learn to heal people and places and things and events that are not there in front of you!

Also from Reiki 3 onwards, you will be able to know where the problem is when a person complains of ailment.

In Reiki 4, you will know about basic anatomy as it is very much necessary to heal the physical body of a person. Also, you will learn many different ways to detect the problem area and heal it.

Once you master all these 4 levels, if you feel that you wish to learn how to attune and teach this wonderful method to others, you may learn further 6 levels that will make you a Reiki teacher, a Reiki grandmaster and a Reiki great grand master.

Of course, learning teachers' levels is never so easy like learning this first level of Reiki, as in these levels, a very deep cleansing of the inner self happens and once this is done, you are taught the methods of teaching as well as attuning at various levels.

Anyways, let us now start with the basic introduction to Reiki and move further with the speed you choose. Here in the first level, we learn how Reiki originated, and what must be our mindset while healing with Reiki, and how we can heal by touch.

INTRODUCTION

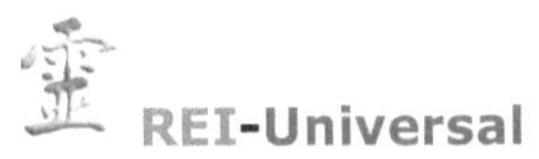 **REI-Universal**   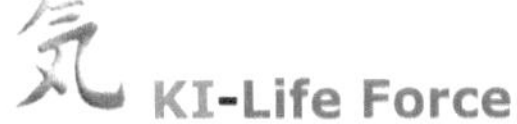 **KI-Life Force**

Reiki is the universal life force that exists everywhere. We experience its presence at all the times. Different people call it by different names & know it in different forms. This energy runs the whole universe. It is **LOVE OF GOD ALIVE**! It is just there irrespective of recognition or imagination as sun, moon & air that are present everywhere. **IT IS ABOVE ALL RELIGIONS**!

Our body systems are designed to have an access to this force. This is the reason why whenever we have any pain, we automatically place our hand over the paining area. Our body mechanism is designed to heal by placing the hand over the ailing area, just as the systems of animals are designed to heal their ailing area by licking it continuously!

Due to our ignorance, we are not able to establish this access. Due to disuse, many people also lose this ability to establish connection with this energy. This is why though simple to use, many cannot use this energy in their daily routine. To regain this wonderful power we need to undergo a complete training and have the connection to this power restored during this training by a simple procedure known as attunement that is given as a part of Reiki training. This is where the Reiki teacher comes into picture.

A Reiki teacher re-establishes the contact of the student with the universal life force by way of a process known as attunement or initiation. This process lets you access this universal life force and even transmit it to others for healing. As one is attuned, one may have some unique experiences. These vary from person to person. But that does not make this science objective and imaginary. The Reiki attunement enables you to heal not to initiate. But Reiki healer finds the transformed life!

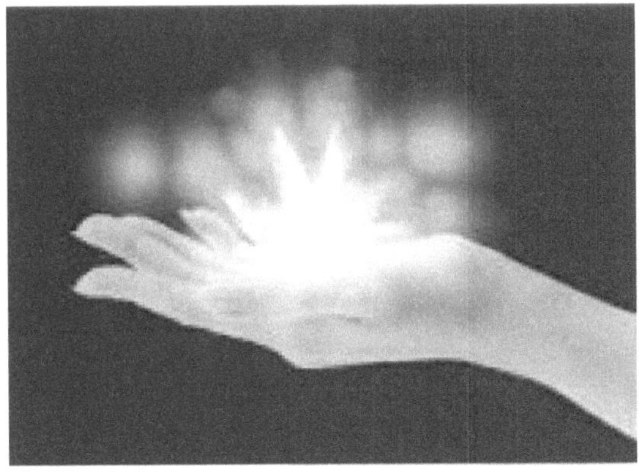

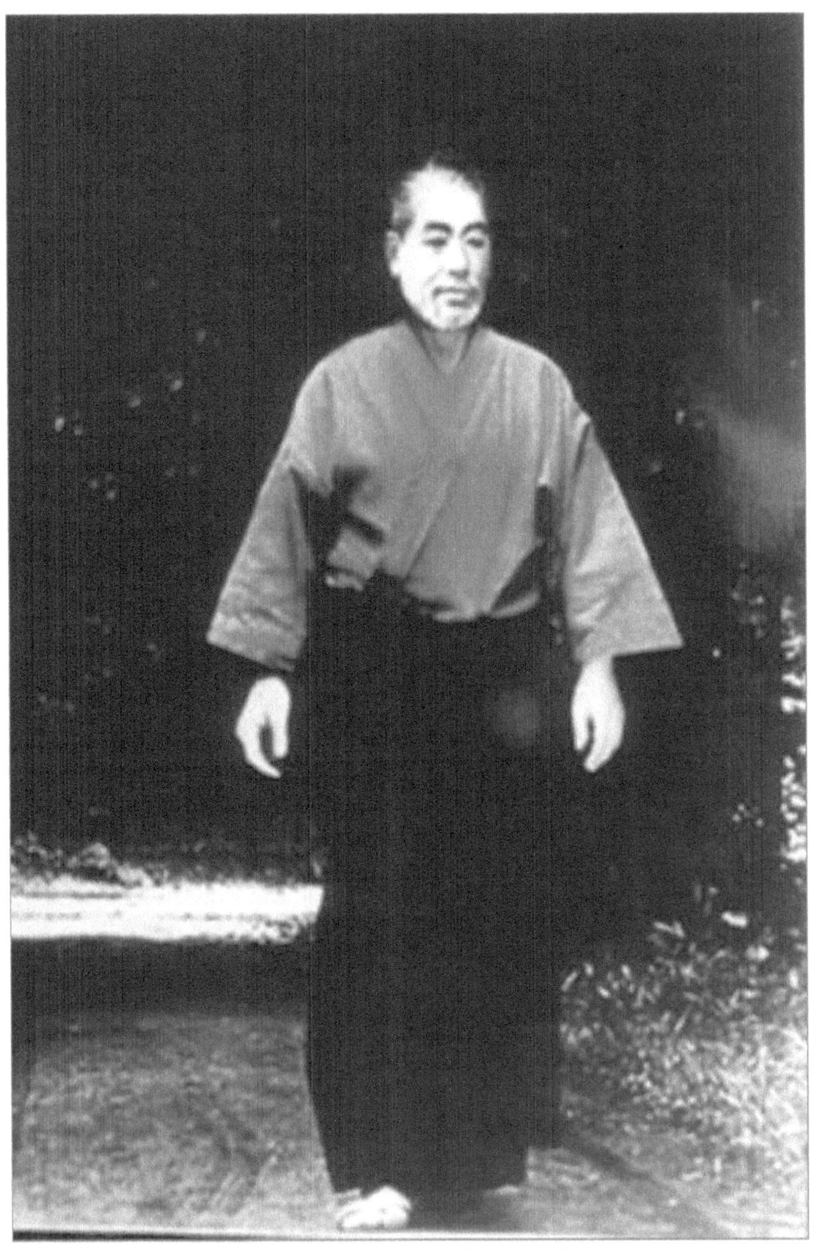

DR. MIKAO USUI
FOUNDER OF REIKI

Reiki is a science of an Indian origin, rediscovered by a Japanese priest, **Dr. Mikao Usui**. In April 1922, **Mikao Usui** opened his first **'Spiritual Seat of Learning'** in Harajuku Tokyo. His teachings were what are called a **'Ronin' (leaderless) method**, this was to ensure that no one-person could lay claim to them, then, or in the future. This would keep them freely available for all who wanted to practice.

Usui was an admirer of the literary works of the **Emperor Meiji** (明治天皇 *Meiji tennō*). While in the process of developing his Reiki system, Usui summarised some of the emperor's works into a set of ethical principles, which later became known as the **Five Reiki Precepts** (五戒 *Gokai*, meaning "The Five Commandments", from the Buddhist teachings against killing, thievery, sexual misconduct, lying, and intemperance).

He not only practiced and taught his Spiritual Teachings but also gave healing. From what we now understand of the way he worked, it seems very possible that he was accepted by his Buddhist leaders as a teacher.

He was often accompanied by Buddhist monks/nuns and also until about eighteen months before he died his teachings were given only to Buddhist and Shinto followers.

He made no provision for his teachings to be continued after his death. He had expected others to come along who would surpass his own capabilities, this did not happen. Curiously Dr. Usui never used the term Reiki for his healing. The term 'Reiki' may have been introduced by Hayashi or the **Gakkai**. The name used by Usui's students is **'Usui Do'** or **'Usui Teate'**. **Hayashi's disciples from U.S.A** *spread the name* **Reiki.**

The popular story about the origin of Reiki is, Dr. Usui believed in answering all questions of his disciples. One disciple asked about the method involved in the touch healing used in Christian faith healing.

He did not have the answer. He said he will find out. He went on searching for it. He searched through Japan & china. On finding nothing satisfactory there, he came to India, studied Sanskrit, & some scripts. Then he went to Tibet to study more Buddhist scripts. Here he found PADMA-SUTRAS from PAUSHKAR-SAMHITA (the book on charkas or Body-Lotuses) called Lotus Sutras by the Reiki people. Then he meditated on the mountain Kurama in Kyoto, got enlightenment and got Reiki.

Kurama is also a very special place for Martial Arts; it is the abode of the Tengu who impart the secrets of Budo to worthy warriors. Morihei Usheiba, founder of Aikido often took students to the mystical Shojobo Valley to train. Despite what the memorial states it was not usual for this sort of meditation to have been taken on Kurama. However it is recorded that this occurred, but it was very late in his life and long after he had started teaching. In the records, no special event is recorded. In traditional western Reiki a great deal of importance is put on the Kurama story, however, this is not true and not referred to by his students.

No evidence is known of his ever being taught in any way by Christian teachers / ministers. He never had any medical training and was never referred to as 'doctor'. This information comes from 'living' students of Mikao Usui some of them are also his relatives. In 1923 shortly before noon on 1st. September, an earthquake shook Tokyo and Yokohama. Over 100,000 deaths were reported. It was the greatest natural disaster in Japanese history. Mikao Usui with his helpers took his healing to the area and as a result of his work became very famous.

During this emergency Usui Sensei's way of giving relief was to 'reach out his hands of love to suffering people'. It is quite possible that as he was living & working in the Tokyo area that his school /home may have been directly affected by the earthquake. *Following the earthquake he was awarded an honorary 'Doctorate of Literature', this was in recognition of his services to the public during the emergency.*

In the last year of his life, the Naval Commanders - Ushida, Taketomi, Hayashi and others, approached him & asked him to teach them. They only learned his healing method. For them he introduced the term 'Ryuku' which means, someone who is a good practitioner but not familiar with the full teachings. There was no formal teaching structure. 'Usui-sensei told that his method is a spiritual healing technique and an energy healing technique. Spiritual healing brings fundamental healing by helping us to become part of the universal consciousness, while energy healing centres on removing the symptoms of mind and body disorders.'

Mikao Usui (1865.8.15-1926.3.9) 臼井甕男 was born on August 15, 1865 in the village of Taniai 合谷 in the Gifu district of Japan. In 1920s he developed a spiritual system based on ancient Taoist practices but uniquely Japanese in style. Usui died from a stroke in a town called on March 9, 1926 in Fukuyama in Hiroshima - Ken.

PEOPLE WHON TOOK REIKI TO THE REST OF THE WORLD:

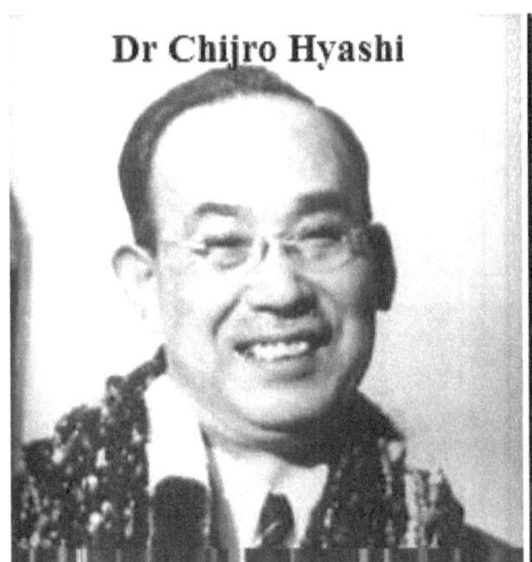

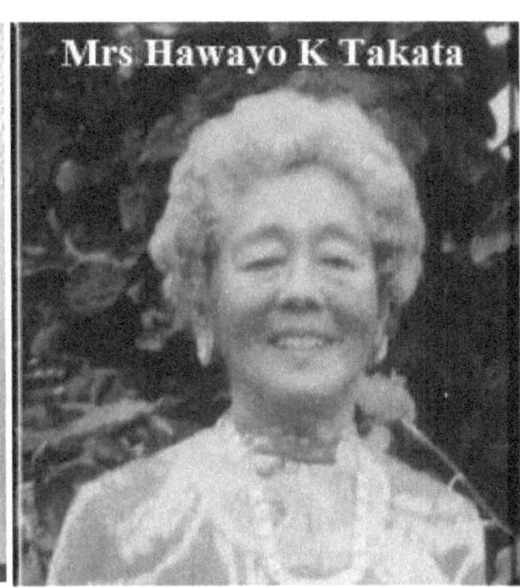

DR. CHIJIRO HAYASHI & MRS. HAWAYO TAKATA

REIKI-1

WHAT YOU LEARN IN REIKI-1

In **SHUYOKAI** i.e. Reiki-1, **Shoden** ("初伝" in Japanese, meaning "Elementary/Entry Teachings") we learn to heal by touch. Also we get to know about this wonderful science that is so simple. The principles of Reiki let you lead your life more powerfully if followed rightly. The rules of Reiki help you be on the ground in spite of generating this wonderful power to change your life as well as the lives of others and the nature.

Reiki 1 begins with the introduction and history of Reiki.

Then you learn the **GOKAI** i.e. Principles of Reiki. These are supposed to be practiced in your daily routine.

After learning the principles, a student learns Rules of Reiki that tell you the dos & don'ts, of Reiki that are to be practiced every time one is giving Reiki to ones own self or to anyone else.

Once he learns this well, he learns the principle behind touch healing. Then he learns how to place hands for healing. Then he learns about the most receptive points of healing in the body. Now he learns about how and how long one must place the hands for healing.

He practices this healing before attunement. This enables him to know the feelings in the hands before attunement. Now the student is attuned into Reiki 1.

After attunement, he has to practice healing again to know the difference in the feeling in hands before and after attunement.

Then the teacher gives some concluding tips and tells the student about the areas in life where he can use this healing method. The teacher also tells the student to experiment freely and use this wonderful method in as many ways as he can. Normally, a master teacher also tells the student to practice regularly at least for 21 days. This is just to make sure that the student uses Reiki well. Also the Reiki teacher tells the student to feel free to ask for any support in the Reiki matter anytime he needs.

PRINCIPLES OF REIKI

While practicing Reiki, a Reiki practitioner is expected to follow some principles in daily life. These were given by the founder of Reiki, Dr. Mikao Usui as a method of life that every Reiki practitioner must bring in practice. He called these principles as **Gokkai**.

Usui was an admirer of the literary works of the **Emperor Meiji** (明治天皇 *Meiji tennō*). While in the process of developing his Reiki system, Usui summarised some of the emperor's works into a set of ethical principles, which later became known as the **Five Reiki Precepts** (五戒 *Gokai*, meaning "The Five Commandments", from the Buddhist teachings against killing, thievery, sexual misconduct, lying, and intemperance).

Of course, they are good even in everyday life for all & mostly taught to all in morals class. As many other principles, these too are easy to preach & difficult to practice.

But I have tried to explain them in such a way that their practice can be practical, logical and easier.

These principles are:

1. *JUST FOR TODAY, I WILL NOT GET ANGERY.*
2. *JUST FOR TODAY, I WILL NOT BE WORRIED.*
3. *JUST FOR TODAY, I WILL BE HONEST IN LIFE.*
4. *JUST FOR TODAY, I WILL LOVE & RESPECT ALL.*
5. *JUST FOR TODAY, I WILL BE THANKFUL TO ALL.*

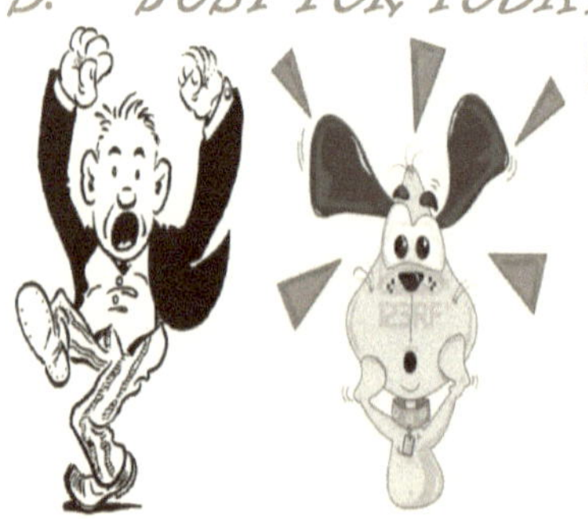
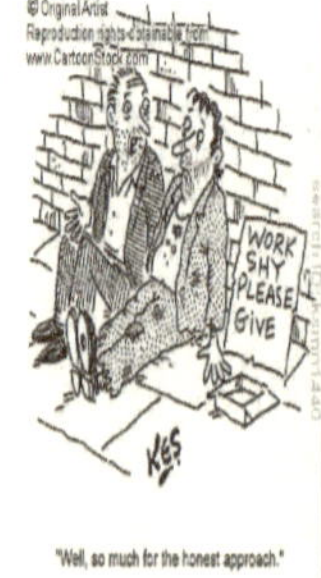
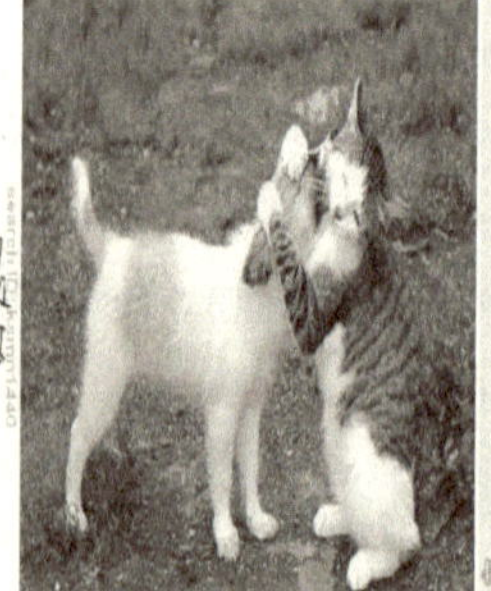

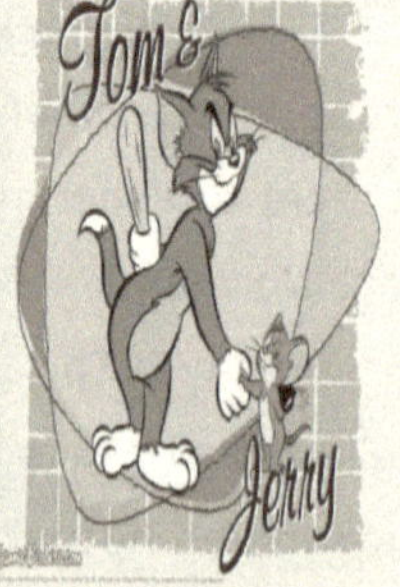

JUST FOR TODAY, I WILL NOT GET ANGERY:

This principle says that one must never get angry with others. The reason behind this is that when one feels helpless and defeated, the ego of a person tries the last resort of overcoming the situation by threatening the person who is causing the state of helplessness or defeat by trying to threaten him through a temper tantrum.

But in fact this comes as a loud declaration of your defeat and helplessness. Due to this if anyone is deliberately trying to harm you, he will know that all your defences are over. As a result, he will harm you more. When you know that anger is a loud declaration of your helplessness, you will never be angry. Of course, the best act in such situation is to keep cool and wait for the right opportunity to handle the situation.

Use anger as a weapon as and when necessary, but never let others control your emotions and be angry to express your helplessness. This means, you can **EXPRESS ANGER** when others understand only the language of anger, but you must **NEVER BE ANGRY** from within! In this way you will learn to use anger like a weapon as & when necessary. You will also learn to protect yourself from being controlled by others!

So, remember that,
ANGER IS A LOUD DECLARATION OF YOUR DEFEAT AND HELPLESSNESS THAT CAN RUIN YOU IF DETECTED BY YOUR OPPONENT & USED BY HIM AGAINST YOU.

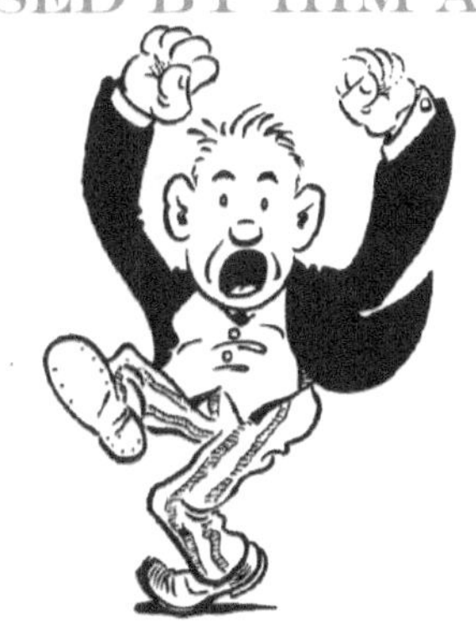

JUST FOR TODAY, I WILL NOT BE WORRIED.

This principle says that one must never worry. Many times people say that one does not worry consciously. The worry automatically happens! But regarding this, you must first understand what happens when you worry.

When we fear the unwanted event and suspect that it will occur, we resist it. Then again we fear its occurrence and resist it again. When this process continues, we say that we are worrying. In fact every time when we imagine the unwanted event, we become instrumental in bringing it into reality. The more we imagine it the more we bring it to reality. This way, by worrying actually we create the event we fear.

Once you know this reality about worry, you will never dare to worry! But you must know what to do at such times. The solution is a very easy. Just prepare yourself to face the event!

So, remember, that
WORRY IS A PASSIVE RESISTANCE TO THE ANTICIPATED UNWANTED EVENT THAT WEAKENS YOU, WHEREAS, TAKING CARE IS AN ACTIVE PREPARATION TO HANDLE THE ANTICIPATED UNWANTED EVENT THAT STRENGTHENS YOU AND LETS YOU HANDLE THE POSSIBLE PROBLEM AS WELL AS THE ANXIETY BUILT DUE TO ITS POSSIBILITY.

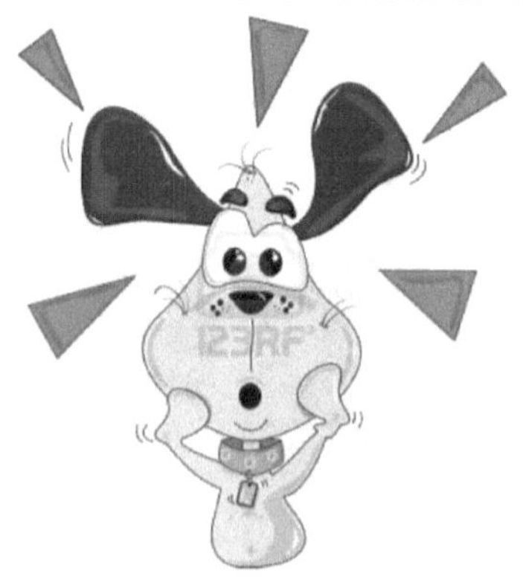

JUST FOR TODAY, I WILL BE HONEST IN LIFE.

This principle says that one must always be honest. Being honest does not just mean speaking the truth and doing things in the right and truthful way. It also means to be truthful to ones own self. For example, many a times we say that we have to do something against our wish.

This time, we are not honest with ourselves. We are deceiving ourselves to save our ego. In fact, when we do anything, we are doing it with our own choice. But at times, when we choose our desired thing, the thing that accompanies it is a thing that we want to avoid.

So, to avoid the unwanted thing, we choose a thing that we actually do not want. But this too is our choice. Yet we never recognize it. We say we had to do that thing against our own choice. This is being dishonest with us!

When we understand this, we will really start being honest with ourselves. Then we will stop feeling bad about the things that we feel we have to do against our choice for the sake of others.

This is being honest in the real sense! In the practice of Reiki, it is necessary for a person to be honest in this sense.

This is the honesty which can be defined as follows:

HONESTY GIVES YOU A CLEAR THINKING. THEN YOU STOP PLAYING GAMES WITH YOURSELF. THEN YOU START HEADING TOWARDS BEING A SUCCESSFUL PERSON WHO DARES TO FACE HIMSELF!

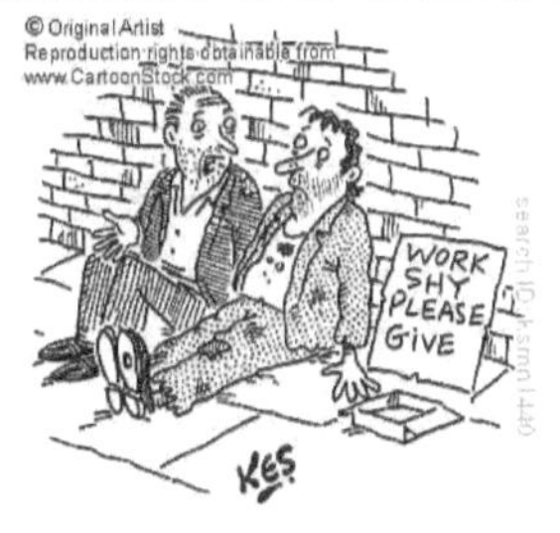

"Well, so much for the honest approach."

JUST FOR TODAY, I WILL LOVE & RESPECT ALL.

This principle teaches you to love and respect all. The word all includes all living and non-living.

The real meaning of this principle is that when we give love and respect, we receive love and respect from universe.

In the universe we always get the same thing that we give. That is why when we give love to all; we also receive it in abundance.

We may or may not receive love and respect from the same persons or things to which we express love.

But we are sure to receive it from many other directions. This is because when we express love and respect to all, we become an expression of love and respect.

LOVE AND RESPECT TO ALL MAKES YOU RESPECTABLE AND LOVABLE IN THE EYES OF OTHERS.

REMEMBER ALL INCLUDES YOU TOO.

SO YOU HAVE TO LOVE AND RESPECT YOURSELF ALONG WITH ALL THINGS AND PERSONS YOU LOVE AND RESPECT.

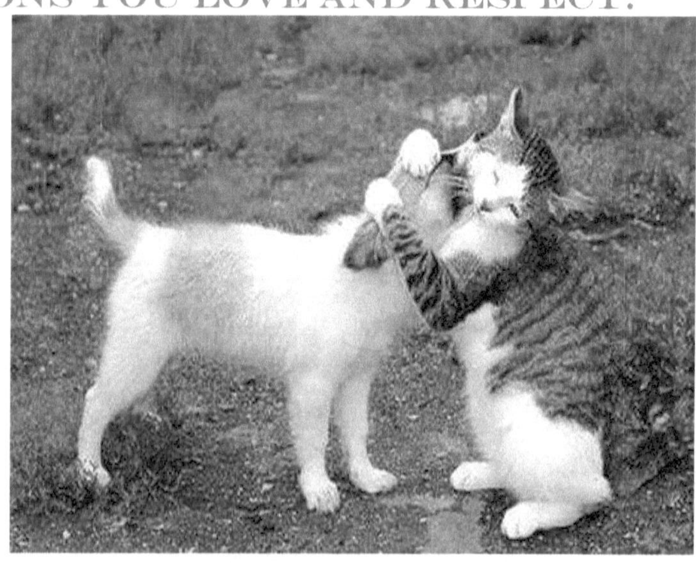

JUST FOR TODAY I WILL BE THANKFUL TO ALL.

This principle teaches you to be thankful to all. It says that we must become the living expressions of gratitude. We keep receiving so many things from so many people and things around us, but hardly do we recognize them!

Are we thankful to the nature for giving us fresh air and water and food? Are we thankful to the Sun for giving us the light? Are we thankful to mother earth for letting us be on it? Are we thankful to our parents for bringing us in this beautiful world? Are we thankful to our teachers for making us capable of earning today? Are we thankful to our kids for choosing us as parents? But unfortunately, we have learned to find faults & blame more perfectly than to thank!

Anyway, if that's our upbringing we need not prove its perfection by blaming it! We can still train ourselves to thank those who have helped us in some or the other way. But when we think of the persons who have harmed us what do we do? Naturally, we say that we cannot thank them. We also ask why of all we must thank those who have harmed us! The answer is very simple. Every event as well as act has two sides, good and bad. The one that appears first in front of us is mistaken to be having only that quality.

In fact we must know that every good event has a bad side in it and every bad event has a good side in it. It is up to us to choose the side of each event.

IF WE DEVELOP A HABIT TO FIND OUT AND ACCEPT ONLY THE POSITIVE SIDE OF EACH EVENT, NOTHING CAN HARM US, AT THE SAME TIME; WE GET THE ABILITY TO CONVERT ANY BAD EVENT INTO GOOD ONE!

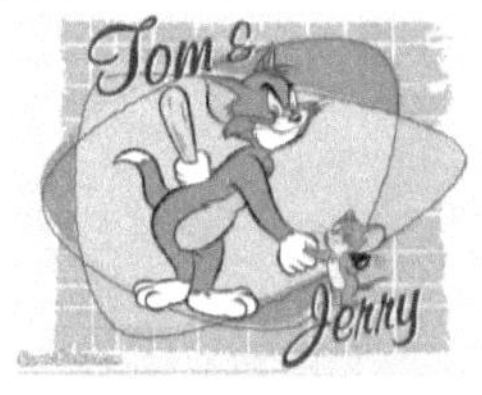

ORIGINAL PRINCIPLES AS GIVEN BY DR. MIKAO USUI
Romaji

招福の秘法
萬病の霊薬
今日丈けは　怒るな
心配すな　感謝して
業をはげめ　人に親切に
朝夕合掌して心に念じ
口に唱へよ
心身改善　臼井霊気療法
肇祖
臼井甕男

<u>**Japanese Pronunciation**</u>

Shou fuku no hiihou
Manbyou no Rei yaku
Kyo dake wa Ikaruna
Shinpai suna Kansha shite
Gyo wo hageme Hito ni shinsetsu ni
Asa yuu gassho shite kokoro ni neji
Kuchi ni tonaeyo
Shin shin kaizen, Usui Reiki Ryoho
Chosso
Usui Mikao

Literal Translation

We are Inviting blessings of the secret method.
Many illnesses of the spiritual (heavenly) medicine
Today only anger not.
Worry not. Be with appreciation.
Do work. To people be kind.
In morning at night hands held in prayer think in your mind
Chant with mouth
Mind body change it for better Usui Reiki method
Founder
Usui Mikao

BENEFITS OF PRACTICE OF PRINCIPLES OF REIKI:

When we start following the above five principles in our daily life, our life will be more beautiful. We will be in a position to get the best out of anything that we get in life.

Then there will be fewer situations to be unhappy about and more situations to be happy about. We can then be a happier person.

This is a situation that everyone longs to have in ones life at all the times! If you study the principles and the explanation about them well, it will be easy for you to make them a part of your being.

This will shift your life to a great new dimension!

This is the reason why Dr. Usui had given great importance to the GOKAI i.e. the principles of Reiki.

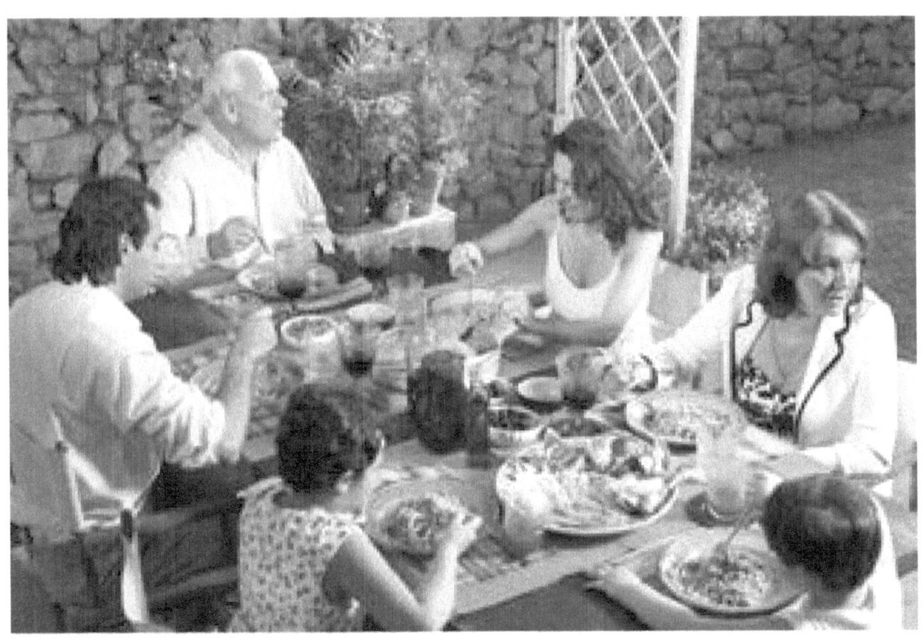

RULES OF REIKI

In the practice of Reiki, we have to avoid certain attitudes when we heal. This helps us to produce a powerful healing with our mind channelled in the right way. While giving Reiki, we must remember these things well.

These are as follows:

1. **DON'T CONSIDER YOURSELF AS A DOCTOR.**
2. **DON'T GIVE REIKI; MAKE IT AVAILABLE.**
3. **DON'T FORCE REIKI ON ANYONE.**
4. **DON'T GIVE REIKI FOR FREE.**
5. **DON'T BE ATTACHED TO THE RESULT.**

DON'T CONSIDER YOURSELF A DOCTOR.

When you are giving Reiki, you are just a channel.

Reiki has its own intelligence. It flows through you. You shouldn't feel that YOU are a doctor healing the patient.

Be humble. Let Reiki heal the patient through you!

DON'T GIVE REIKI; MAKE IT AVAILABLE.

When you give Reiki, you are making it available for patient. The body of patient receives the necessary amount of Reiki & heals itself.

Remember; you are not GIVING Reiki, the patient is RECEIVING. You are just making Reiki available to the patient to heal himself.

DON'T FORCE REIKI ON ANYONE.

When someone doesn't want Reiki, don't force it. When a person has said no, he will not receive Reiki even if you try to give.

This is just as when a person has closed the door of his house, you cannot enter the house till the person opens the door!

Similarly when one has said no, you may keep giving Reiki and nothing will happen. At such times keep quiet. Know that the person has chosen the problem by himself so let him be with it!

If you want to help someone but feel that he won't accept Reiki, don't talk about it. Just give Reiki.

If soul of the person is ready, he will receive it. But this can happen only when his conscious mind is neutral!

DON'T GIVE REIKI FOR FREE.

When you are giving anything, the circuit gets completed only after you receive something in exchange.

It is the same principle on which the electricity flows. You must have seen two pins in the electric plug. One is for giving and the other is for receiving.

So, unless and until you don't receive anything in return of Reiki, the Reiki given will not work. This is the reason why this rule is made.

DON'T BE ATTACHED TO THE RESULT.

The law of cause and effect says that if the right cause is created, the right result will automatically be created. We have the power to create the cause. The cause produces result!

Do you know the principle of Karma stated in Bhagwad-Gita?

In one stanza *Lord Krishna* says:

KARMANYEVADHIKARASTE, MA PHALESHU KADACHANA,
MA KARMAPHALAHETURBHU, MA TE SANGOSTVAKARMANI

कर्मण्येवाऽधिकाऽरस्ते मा फलेषु कदाचन
मा कर्मफलहेतुर्भूः मा नं सङ्गोऽस्त्वकर्मणि

Many people interpret this as the theory that tells you to keep doing your work without expecting the result. But this is not so. It says that you have the power (*adhikara*) to produce the action (*karma*), not the result (*phala*). Never try to create (*heturbhu*) the result (*phala*). At the same time, never refrain (*ma te sangostu*) from action (*akarmani*).

This is the most practical explanation about cause and effect relation in nature. We have the power to create the cause that in turn will produce the effect we want. We cannot produce the effect directly.

But we must remember that if our cause is right enough to produce the result, we are sure to get the result in due course. So, we must let the cause produce the result & give it necessary time.

Law of cause says, *if conclusion is wrong, check the premises!*

If the **premises are right, conclusion has to be right**. You don't have to expect it, desire it, want it, or so. It is inevitable and will come to you even if you don't expect desire, want or think about it!

HOW TO HEAL WITH REIKI

The method of healing with Reiki is very simple. What you have to do is just cup your hands with all fingers joined and place them over the area that is ailing.

The energy will get transmitted to that area through your hand and the area will be healed.

As the healing happens, you will feel the vibrations or heat in your hands. This is an indication of the healing.

You need to learn to read your hands for this feeling during your Reiki class. At times the feeling in your hands differs as per the kind of problem prevailing in the related part.

When you keep the hand over any area, initially you may feel nothing.

After some time, you will start feeling the heat or vibrations or coldness or anything like itching or burning.

This means Reiki flow has started towards the related area. This is how you recognize the presence of Reiki.

At this time, even the patient also feels the flow of Reiki.

When you continue to keep your hand over that area for some more time, this feeling will vanish and the hands will appear normal.

At this time, even the patient may also have some similar feeling & when Reiki flow stops the patient also will feel that your hands have become normal.

This happens on its own when the area you are healing has received the necessary amount of energy.

Just as in the washing machine, when the desired level of water is achieved, the inflow of water stops, in the body, when the desired energy level is reached, the flow of Reiki stops.

This is why we say that we cannot make mistakes with Reiki as the Reiki energy has its own intelligence! When one part of body is healed like this, you may move to other area of problem to heal it.

This is how you can heal the whole body yours & others.

In the later pages you will see how you heal the different parts in the body and which body areas are most sensitive to Reiki.

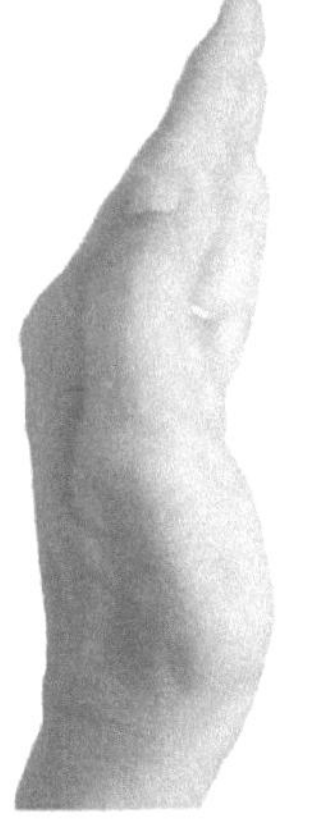
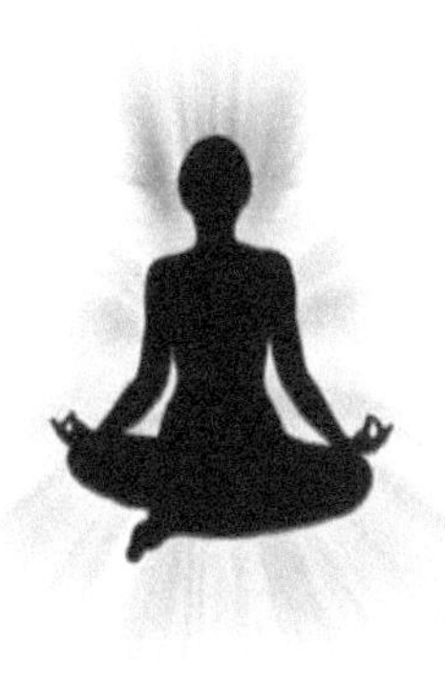
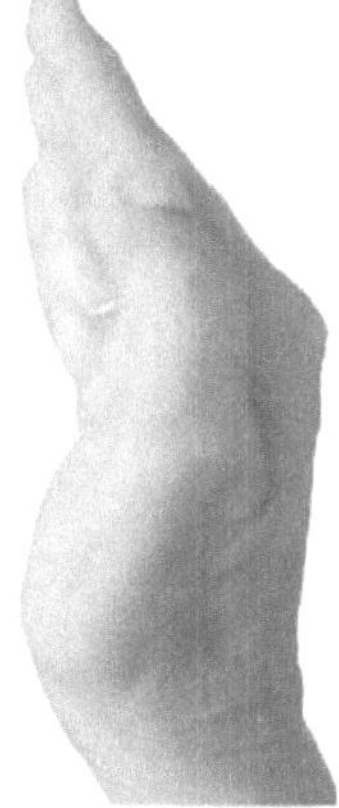

THE ENERGY CENTRES: CHAKRAS:

In our body there are some areas that give and receive energy for the whole body. These are the gateways to the energy for our body. Just as we breathe with our nose, our body energies breathe thro the charkas.

If there is any block in the way of these energies, the body does not receive enough energy, just as when there are clouds in the sky, we do not get good sun light.

Then in the absence of proper energy, the body feels weak & sick. So, the removal of these clouds or blocks is necessary to restore good health. Reiki does this.

So, it is necessary to know the positions of the major charkas before starting with the Reiki training.

The main seven charkas in the body are,

1. **Root Chakra: MULADHARA:** at the tail bone base of spine: governs Physical Awareness, vigour, heredity, survival, security, passion, feet, legs, survival, trust, home, money & job relation.
2. **Sacral Chakra: Swadhisthana:** at sex organs or near belly button: governs anger, fear, social awareness, and sexuality, creativity, emotions, and nurturing, spleen, food or sex perceptions.
3. between the sternum bone & belly: governs Intellectual Awareness, power, accomplishments, will, ego projections, vital energy control, freedom to be oneself.
4. **Heart Chakra: Anahat:** at heart centre of chest: governs Emotions & Security, love, compassion, lungs, breath, Prana, sense of time, relationships in life.
5. **Throat Chakra: Vishuddha:** at base of throat: governs speech, voice, listening, hearing, total self expression, communication, conceptual awareness & ideas.
6. **Third Eye Chakra: Ajna:** in centre of forehead above eyes: governs Intuitive Awareness, intuition, thought, imagination, association of experiences, inner & outer sight, visions, memory, assimilation of perception, dreams.
7. **Crown Chakra: Sahastrara:** Top of head: governs imaginative awareness, connection to cosmic consciousness, spiritual wisdom, desires, true knowledge.

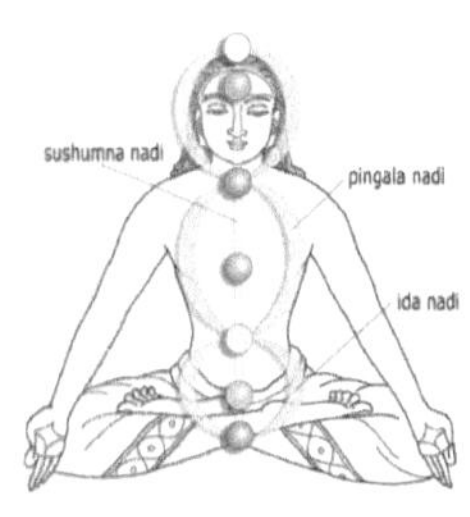

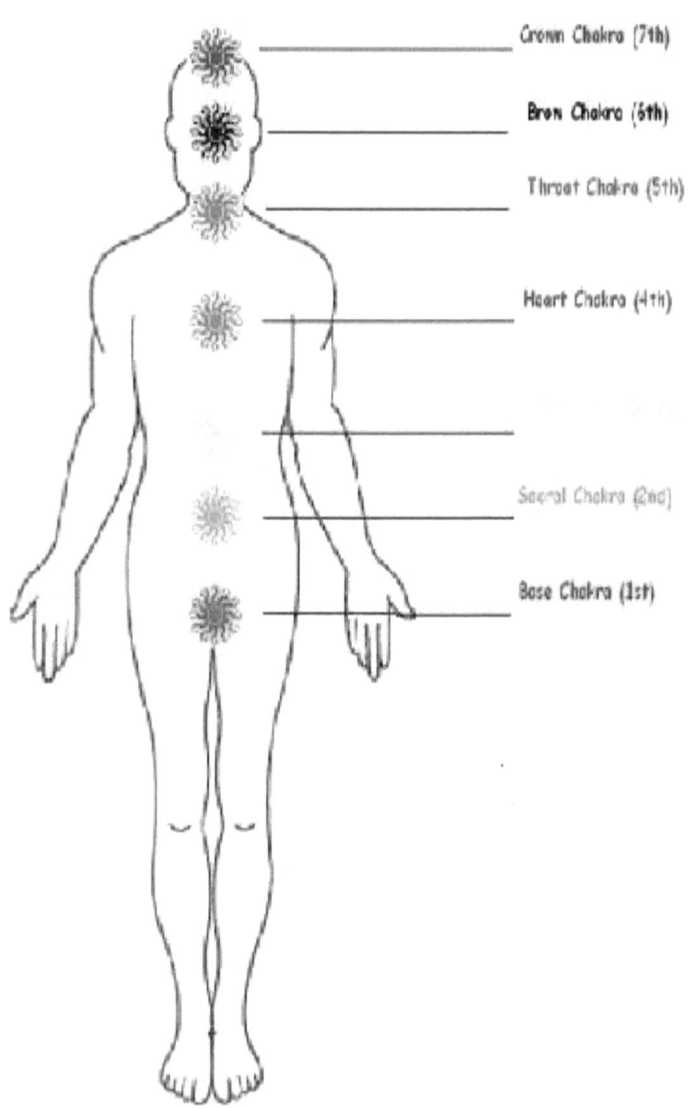

Crown Chakra (7th)
Brow Chakra (6th)
Throat Chakra (5th)
Heart Chakra (4th)
Sacral Chakra (2nd)
Base Chakra (1st)

CHAKRAS (ENERGY CENTRES)

1. **CROWN CHAKRA (PINEAL GLAND)**

   Dark violet.
   It is the opening to the opening to the universe to the highest consciousness and gives experience about who you are.
   Connects us with spiritual self.
   Connected with upper brain & right eye.

2. **THIRD EYE (PITUITARY GLAND)**

   Dark Blue.
   It is the intuition centre and is for inner wisdom.
   Connected with Autonomic nervous system and hypothalamus.

3. **THROAT CHAKRA (THYROID GLAND)**

   Light blue.
   Connected to throat & lungs.
   Function is communication and self expression.

4, **HEART CHAKRA (THYMUS GLAND)**

   Bright light green.
   Connected to heart, lungs, liver & circulatory system.
   Function is live & compassion.

5. **SOLAR PLEXUS (ADRENAL GLANDS)**

   Bright Yellow.
   Connected to stomach, liver & gall bladder.
   Function is Power & Wisdom.
   This is the seat of all emotions and feelings. We draw feelings from Solar Plexus and feel at heart.

6. **HARA /SACRAL CHAKRA (GONADS, TESTICALS & OVARIES)**

   Orange.
   Connected to reproductive organs.
   This is the centre of sexual energy, feelings & emotions.
   Function-Life Centre, create and protect (purpose) life. We can live with ourselves in Hara.

7. **ROOT CHAKRA (SUPRA RENAL)**

   Red.
   Connected to kidneys, bladder and spine.
   Function-survival issues, Seat of KUNDALINI energy, creative expression & Abundance issues.

CHAKRAS; CONNECTED GLANDS & THEIR FUNCTIONS:

NO.	NAME OF THE CHAKRA	CONNECTED GLAND	FUNCTION
1.	SAHASTRARA (Crown)	PINEAL	Regulates water balance, manages working of glands, controls cerebrospinal fluid and sex desires, and stimulates growth of the nerves.
2.	AJNA (Third Eye)	PITUITARY (Master Gland)	Controls air and space, controls the growth of body, brain power and memory.
3.	VISHUDDHA (Throat)	THYROID & PARATHYROID	Controls air, lungs and heart, temperature regulation and governs energy production through control of calcium.
4.	ANAHAT (Heart)	THYMUS	Acts as a God mother till a child is 12 to 15.
5.		PANCREAS	Control fire and production of digestive juices, sodium and water balance, stress activeness and character building, regulates blood and sugar level.
6.	SWADHISTHANA (Hara)	ADRENALS	Controls APAN VAYU function of all organs below diaphragm and movement of stools and urine.
7.	MULADHARA (Root)	SEX & GONADS	Controls water and phosphorus contents, produces sex hormones.

INNER GRATITUDE:

- Sit in a comfortable position.
- Close your eyes.
- Think of all who helped you.
- Think of the benefit you got out of the help.
- Thank them.
- Think of all those who harmed you.
- Find the benefit you got through that harm.
- Thank them.
- Think of those whom you helped.
- Find the benefit you got out of that help.
- Thank them.
- Think of those whom you harmed.
- Mentally ask forgiveness for the harm you did.
- Think of benefits both of you got from the harm.
- Thank them for tolerating you.
- Think of the natural resources that contributed.
- Thank them.
- Feel the gratitude everywhere.
- Find yourself thankful to all the creation of god.
- Slowly open your eyes & start your routine.

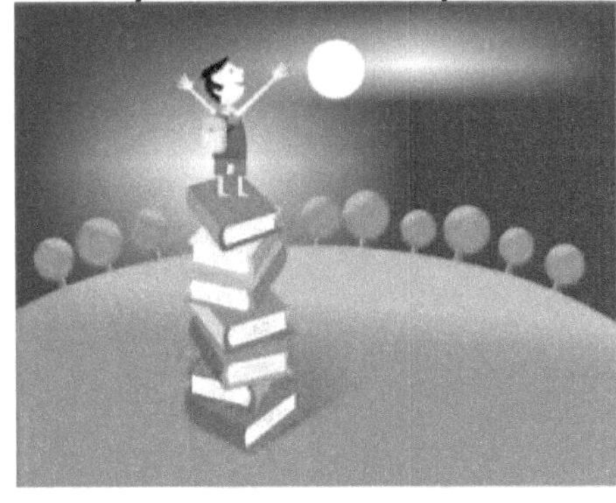

GROUNDING:

- Sit in a comfortable position.
- Close your eyes.
- Concentrate on your breathing.
- Be aware of the energies around.
- Be aware of your thoughts.
- Find the thoughts that make you comfortable.
- Find the thoughts that make you restless.
- Know that restlessness is due to non-grounding.
- Let the divine love shower on you.
- Let these energies enter through top of head.
- Let these energies fill your body.
- Feel the comfort with these energies.
- Let the disturbing thought develop energy roots.
- Let these roots go into the ground.
- Request these roots to reach problem solution.
- Feel the relief from the upsets.
- Now let the divine love create total rooting.
- Feel perfectly grounded with practical attitude.
- Slowly open your eyes and start the routine

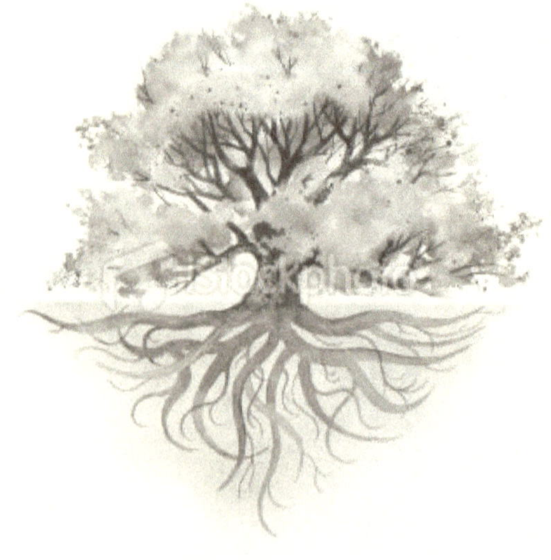

NAADBRAHMA MEDITATION:

- Sit with spine straight & legs folded.
- Concentrate on breathing for a while.
- Keep the mouth closed & close eyes.
- Start the 'hum' sound with exhalation.
- Feel the relaxation with each 'hum'.
- When relaxed, bring palms on naval.
- Let the open palms face upward under naval.
- Continue with 'hum' for some time.
- Feel the energy in and around.
- Spread the palms to shower the energy around.
- With hands on naval, say 'hum' for some time.
- Let the open palms face downwards now.
- Gather the universal energy from around.
- Bring palms on naval and place it in your naval.
- Feel the give and take of energy with universe.
- Lie down on your back with eyes closed.
- Feel the oneness with the universe for a while.
- Find yourself ready for the energy work.
- Slowly open the eyes & start the routine.

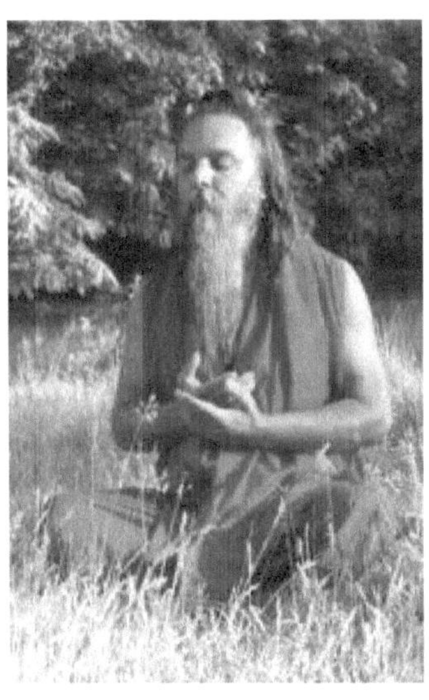

GOLDEN BALL EXERCISE:

- Sit in a comfortable position.
- Close your eyes.
- Visualize the Reiki energy as a golden ball.
- Let it enter your system thro' your crown charka.
- Let this golden ball energize your crown.
- Now let it travel to your third eye.
- Let this golden ball energize your third eye.
- Now let it travel to your throat.
- Let this golden ball energize your throat.
- Now let it travel to your heart.
- Let this golden ball energize your heart.
- Now let it travel to your solar plexus.
- Let this golden ball energize your solar plexus.
- Now let it travel to your sacral chakra.
- Let this golden ball energize your sacral chakra.
- Now let it travel to your root.
- Let this golden ball energize your root.
- Feel the energy of the golden ball in your body.
- Now let the golden ball travel to sacral chakra.
- Let the golden ball settle here.
- Feel full of energy & readiness to heal.
- Open your eyes and start the healing work.

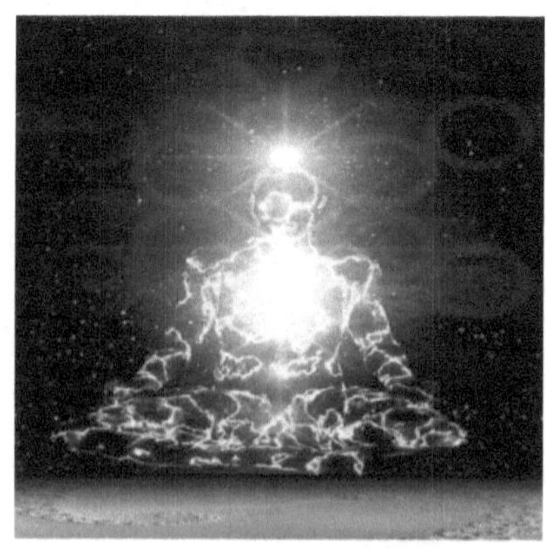

TREATMENT METHOD

Reiki treatment is given to all **PHYSICAL, MENTAL, EMOTIONAL** & **SPIRITUAL** level problems.

In the advanced levels, we may treat the nature, events, thoughts, machines and many similar things. We can even go beyond space & time and treat the past as well as future events. To treat these, we energize the most receptive points of body.

Following steps are followed by many traditional teachers of Reiki; for touch healing as well as complete distance healing of a patient in the later stages, after mentally being grateful to Reiki, the patient & one self:

@ Let the patient lie down on his back.
@ Place your hands on each of the following points for about three to five minutes.
@ Alternately, keep the hands as long as you feel the vibrations & heat in your hands.
@ On the front side, treat the
**EYES,
EARS,
TEMPLES,
FRONT & BACK FOREHEAD,
BACK HEAD,
JAWS,
FRONT & BACK NECK,
SIDES OF NECK,
SHOULDER JOINTS,
UPPER ARMS,
INNER ELBOWS,
OUTER ELBOWS,
FORE ARMS,
WRISTS,
BACK OF PALMS,
PALMS,
LUNG TIPS,
THROAT,
HEART,**

THYROID GLAND,
THYMUS GLAND,
(DIAPHRAGM) SOLAR PLEXUS,
LIVER,
PANCREAS & SPLEEN,
(NAVAL) HARA,
(GROIN) OVARIES or SPERMATIC CORD,
THIGHS,
FRONT KNEES,
BACK KNEES,
LOWER LEGS,
CALF MUSCLES,
ANKLES,
FEET
&
FOOT SOLES.

- Now, With your index and middle finger stretched and rest of the fingers closed, draw anticlockwise spirals to lock the energies given by you, on both the sides simultaneously, around the patient from his head to toes.
- For dong this, hold your hands on both sides of the patient, keeping first two fingers straight and joining ring finger, little finger and thumb, and then move both hands from outward to inward in circles from head to toes of the patient at about 2 inches distance from the body on sides.
- Now ask the patient to turn & lie down on his stomach.
- Start treating the back side.
- Here, treat the

BACK FOREHEAD,
OCCIPITAL LOBE,
SHOULDERS,
BACK THROAT,
BACK SOLAR PLEXUS,
KIDNEYS,
BACK HARA,
BASE OF THE SPINE,
BACK THIGHS,
BACK KNEES,
CALF MUSCLES &
HEELS

- Now, With your index and middle finger stretched and rest of the fingers closed, draw anticlockwise spirals again, to lock the energies given by you, on both the sides simultaneously, around the patient from his head to toes.
- For dong this, hold your hands on both sides of the patient, keeping first two fingers straight and joining ring finger, little finger and thumb, and then move both hands from outward to inward in circles from head to toes of the patient at about 2 inches distance from the body on sides.
- After this, balance the charkas of the patient.
- To balance chakras, place your hands one on each point mentioned below, at about two inches above the point:
- Do this for the following points:
- First place one hand above **back third eye** and the other above the **back root centre**. Check the energies here and move only when both hands have the same kind of vibrations.
- Now move to **occipital lobe** & **back hara**. Place the hands there till energies have the same kind of vibrations.
- Now go to **back throat** & **back solar plexus**. Keep the hands till energies have the same kind of vibrations.
- Now place both hands above **back heart** and keep the hands there till there is even flow of energy.
- This will balance the charkas of the patient.
- This step is necessary to confirm that after healing the energies of the patient are well aligned.
- Now, place the index & middle finger of your right hand on the uppermost part of spine of the patient and forcefully move the fingers quickly down the spine to the base of the spine.
- This concludes the whole body treatment.
- Now you may ask the patient to get up and start his routine.
- Do not forget the post treatment care instructions.
- **Wash your hands thoroughly after treatment.**
- **Change your thoughts to something totally different.**
- Then feel fresh, thank Reiki, and start your routine.

I researched and developed these positions: They are much more than the traditional ones, but work wonders!

REIKI TREATMENT POSITIONS AT A GLANCE:

HEAD	THORAX	BACK	LEGS	HANDS	SIDES
EYES	LUNG TIPS	SHOULDERS	THIGHS	SHOULDER JOINT	UNDER ARMS
EARS	THROAT	B. THROAT	FRONT KNEES	UPPER ARMS	SIDES OF CHEST
TEMPLES	HEART	B. HEART	BACK KNEES	INNER ELBOWS	SIDE OF ABDOMEN
F B FOREHEAD	DIAPHRAGM	B. DIAPHRAGM	LOWER LEGS	OUTER ELBOWS	SIDES OF WAIST
B HEAD	LIVER	KIDNEYS	CALF MUSCLES	FORE ARMS	SIDES OF HIPS
JAWS	SPLEEN	B. NAVAL	ANKLES	WRISTS	SIDES OF THIGHS
F B NECK	NAVAL	WAIST	FEET	BACK OF PALMS	SIDES OF KNEES
SIDES NECK	GROIN	BASE OF SPINE	FOOT SOLES	PALM	SIDES OF ANKLES

Dr. Usui used to heal just on a few points and used to heal the whole body. People feel that since today, the Reiki healers do not have the sane power of healing as Dr. Usui, they must heal ALL the points for total healing. But this is a myth, and in today's hectic life schedule, to find time to heal ALL the above points daily is just next to impossible. So, I am giving the healing points used by Dr. Usui for your reference. They were called "**Head Byosen**".

Here are the healing points that Dr. Usui used for healing:

HEAD BYOSEN: USUI'S ORIGINAL HAND POSITIONS
Healee is seated, not lying down

Healing shall be started from head position.
The following 5 positions shall be healed in 30 minutes total.
Then other required positions showing imbalance are healed.
 (1) Zento-bu:
Forehead top (the line where your hair starts to grow)
(2) Sokuto-bu:
Both sides of your head at the same time
(3) Koutou-bu:
Back of your head and forehead (Nentatsu)
(4) Enzui-bu:
Each side of the neck
(5) Toucho-bu:
Top of your head (crown)
I recommend that you try this method & see what it feels like.
I think we can safely say that following the head Byosen would be practiced for treating any imbalance in body.

REIKI HEALING POSITIONS:

HANDS MUST BE CUPPED AS FOLLOWS WHILE HEALING:

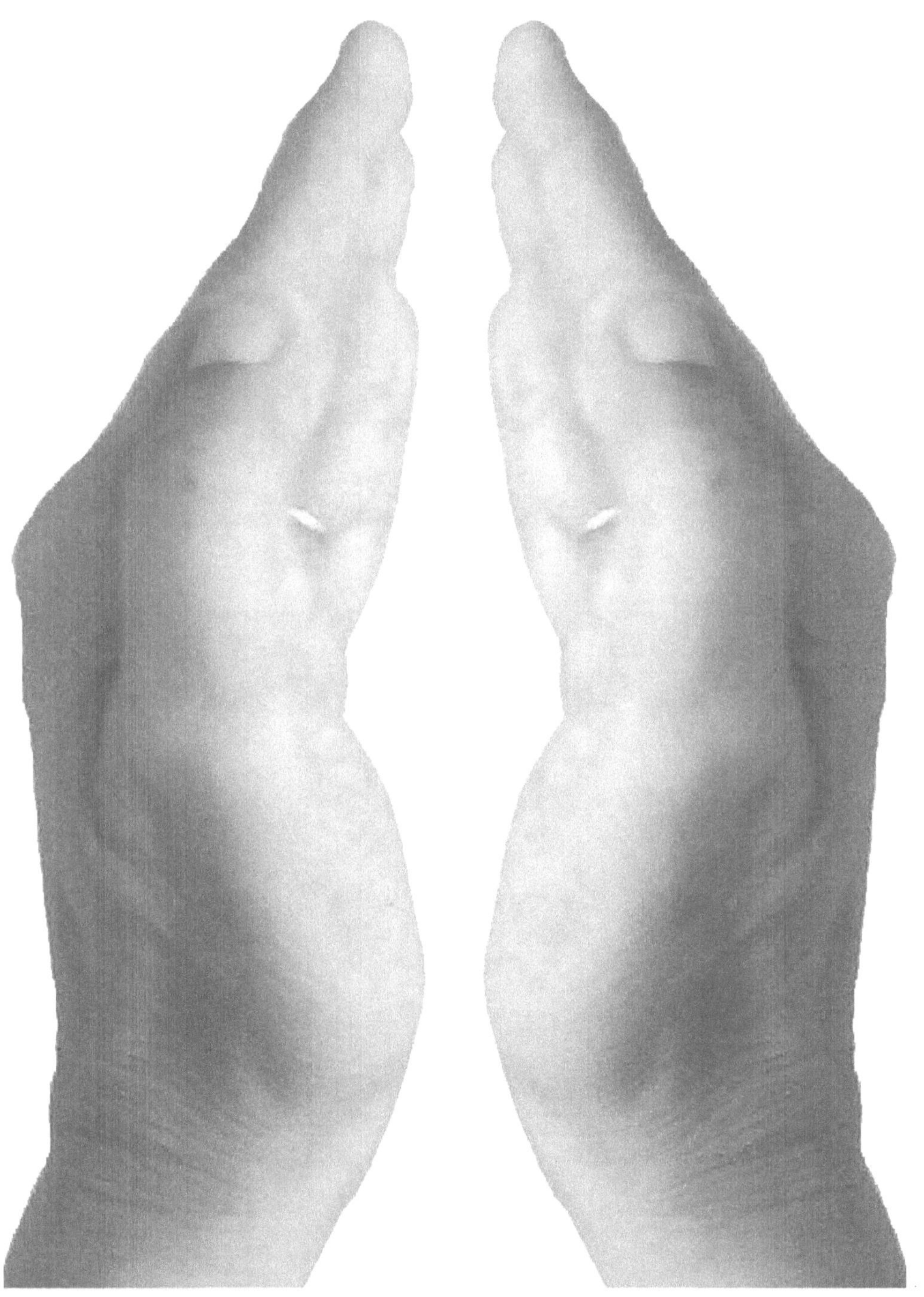

THEN START FEELING THE ENERGY FLOW IN HANDS:

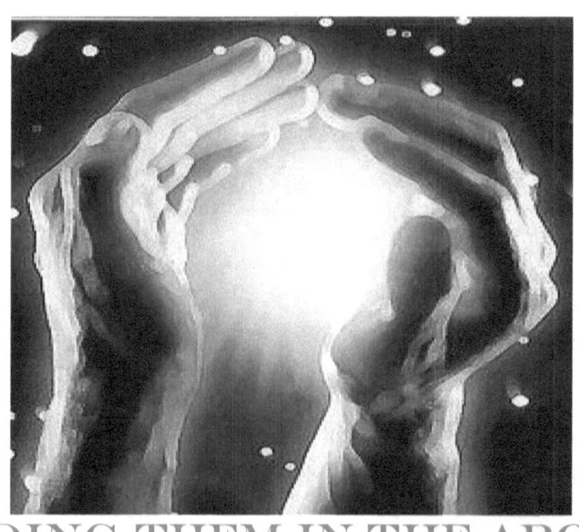

BY HOLDING THEM IN THE ABOVE WAY OR AS:

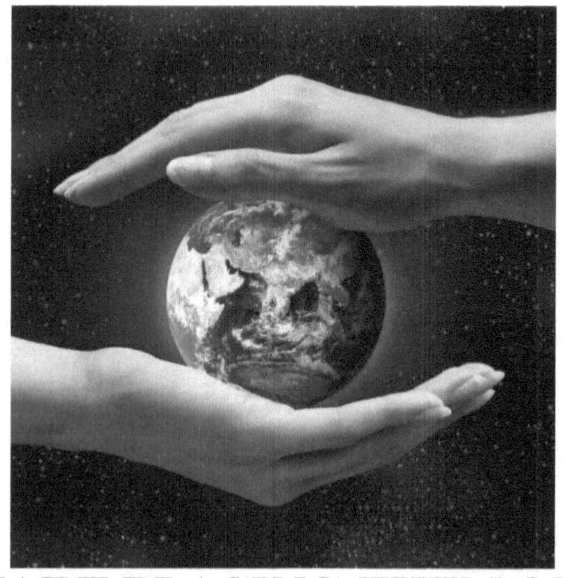

NOW START PLACING THEM ON YOUR BODY AS FOLLOWS:

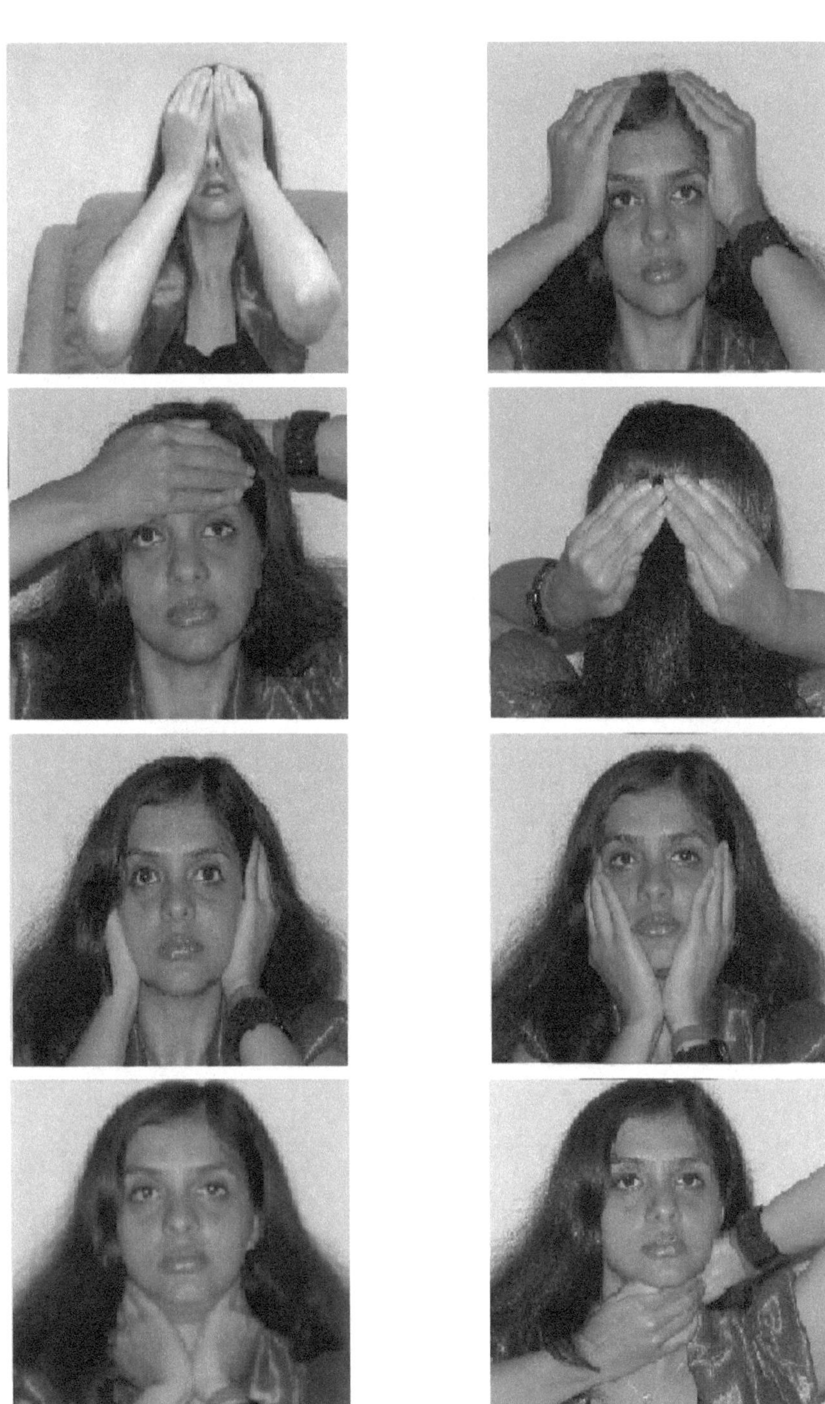

HEAD

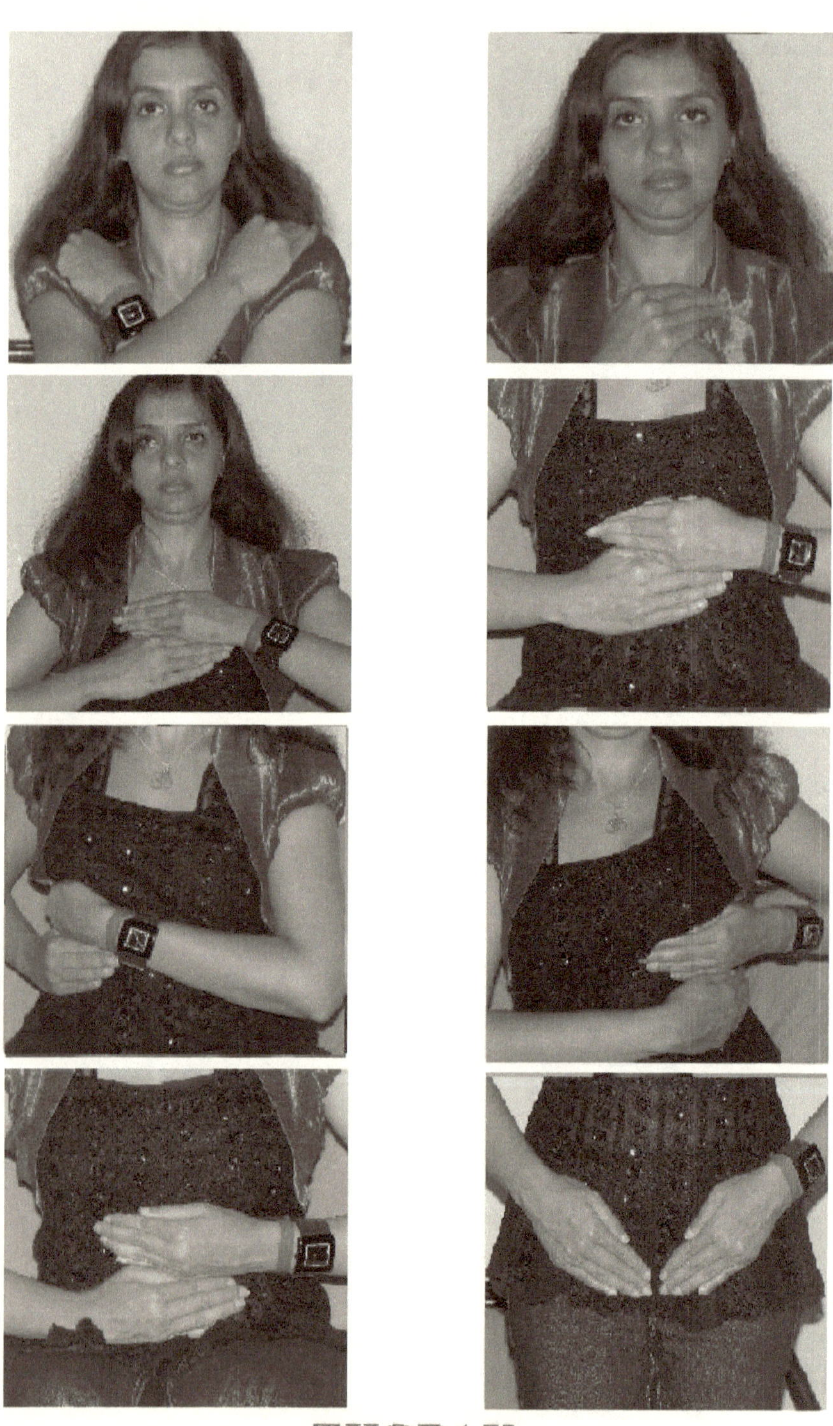

THORAX

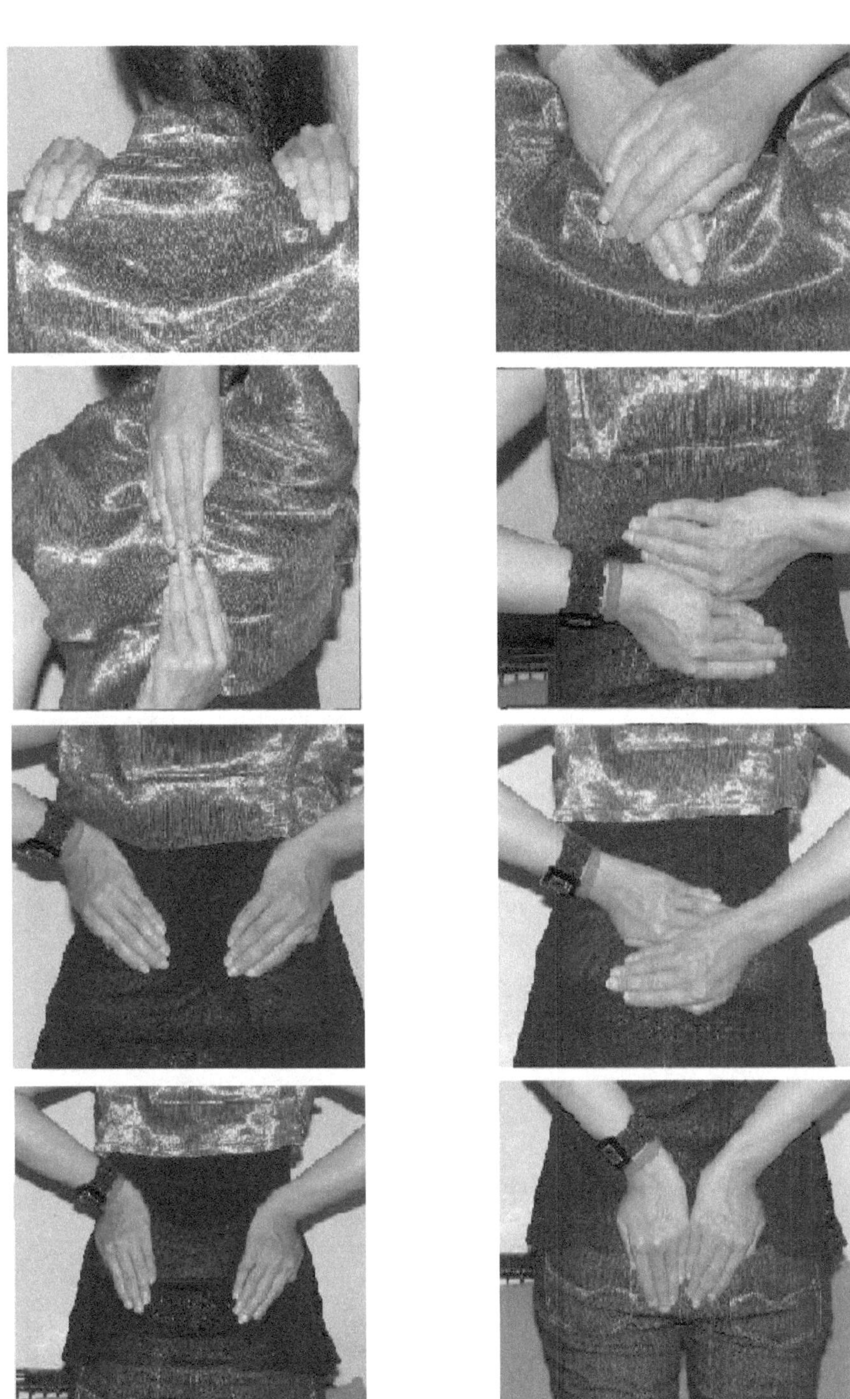

BACK

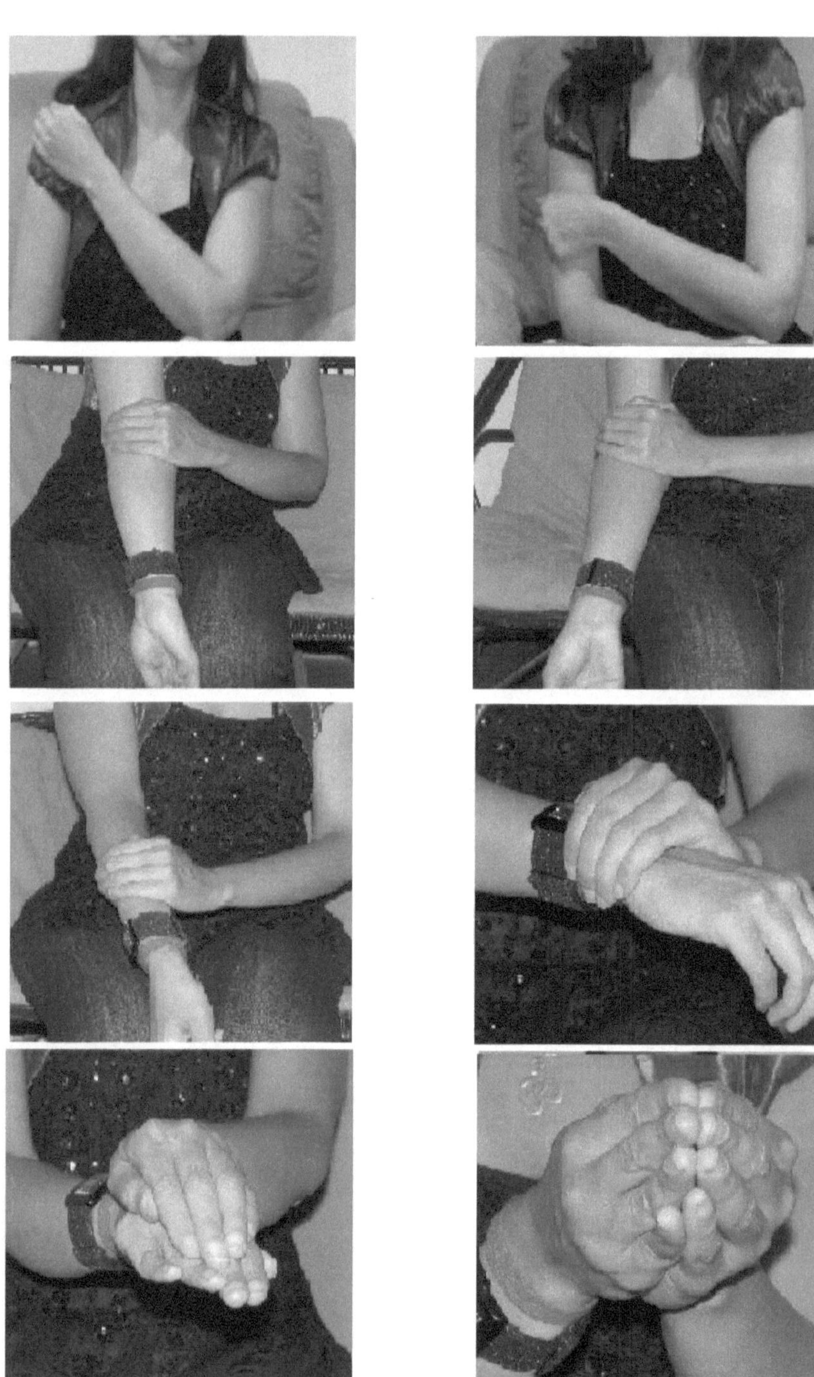

HANDS
RIGHT

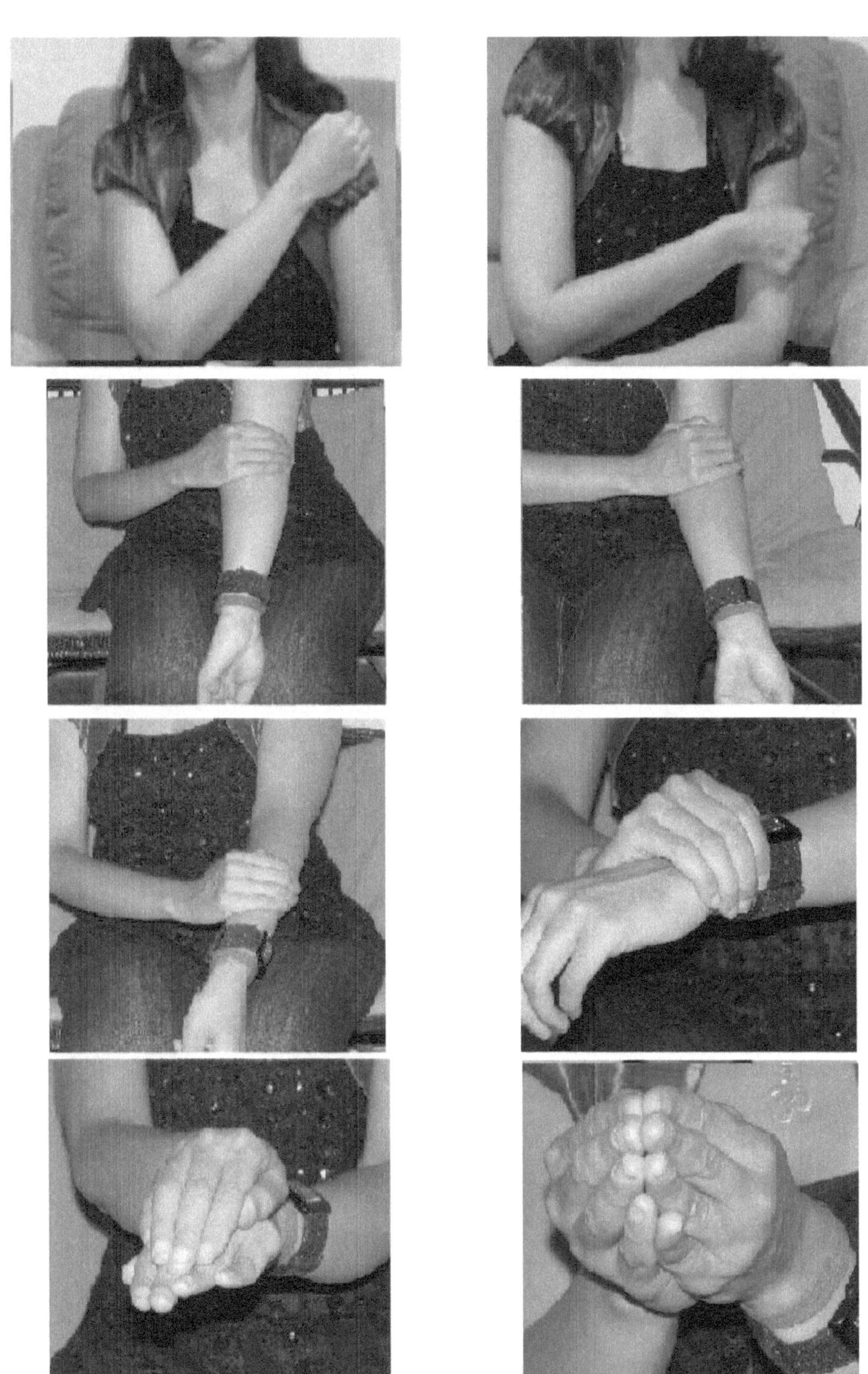

HANDS
LEFT

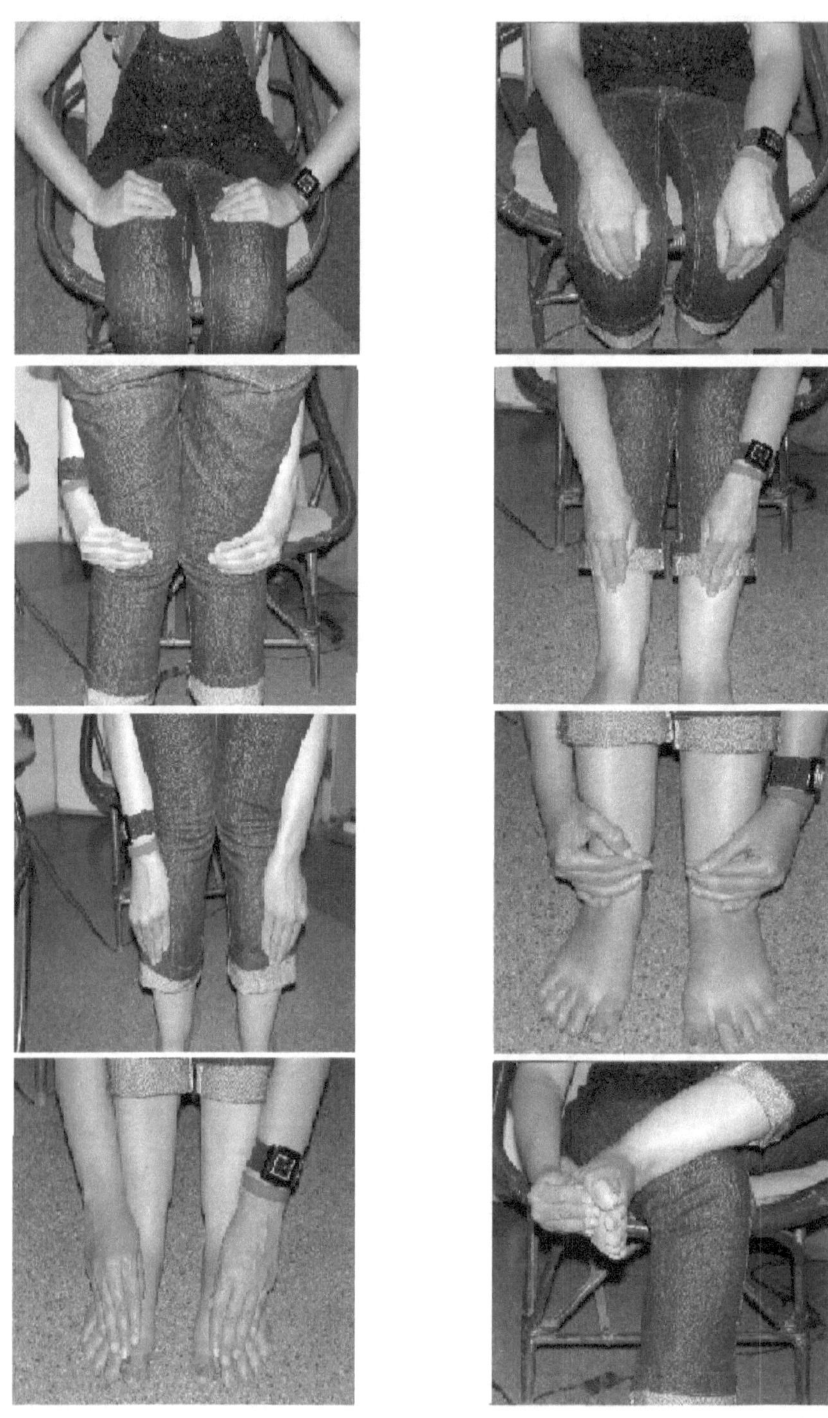

LEGS

59

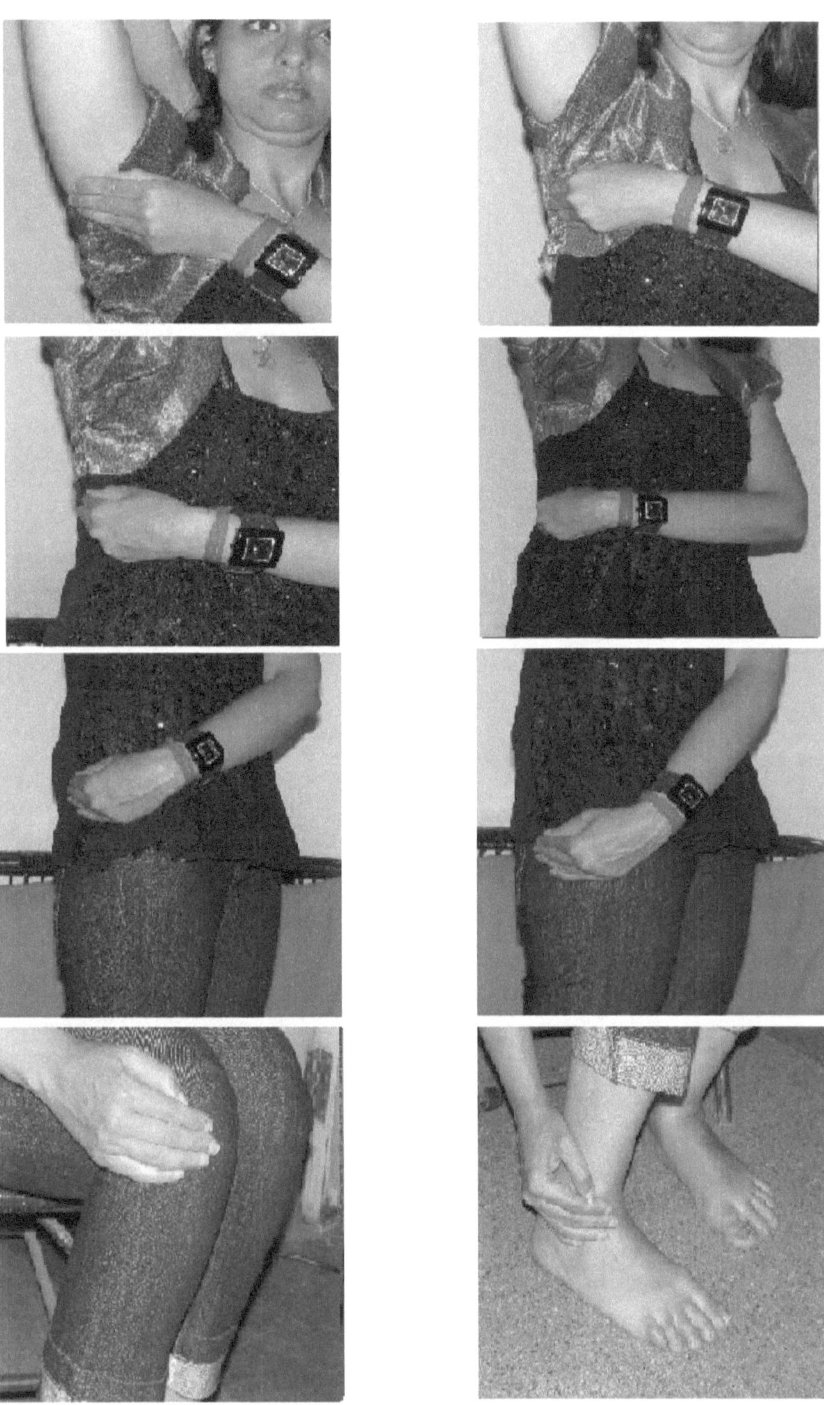

SIDES
RIGHT

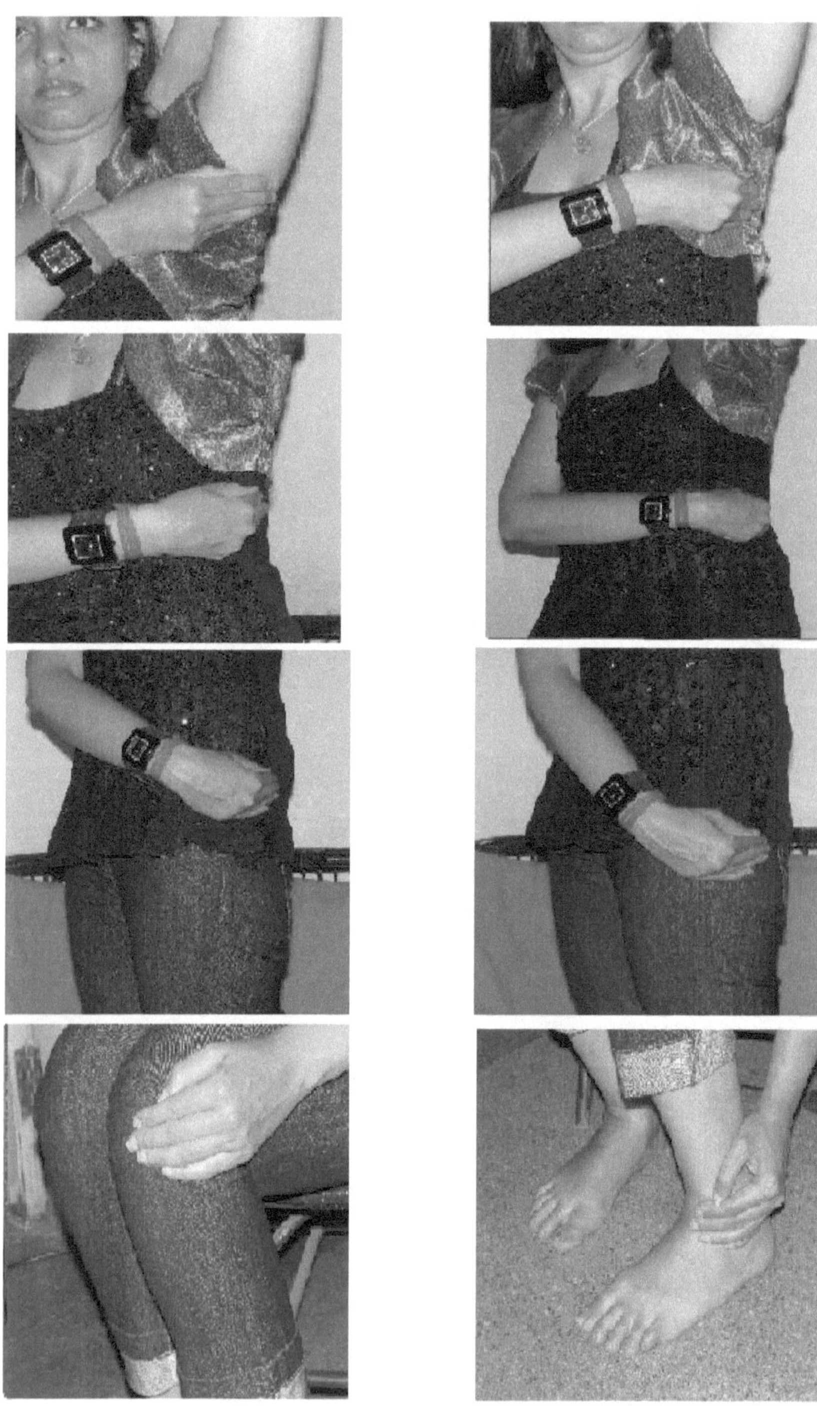

SIDES
LEFT

WHEN NOT TO USE REIKI

- Reiki neutralizes anaesthesia quickly. So do not use Reiki before surgery or dental work.
- Do not use on broken bones until a Doctor has set them. Otherwise bones may join before right placement.
- Do not use on a severed limb until it has been re-attached. The energy can seal off veins and nerves making it hard to re-attach the limb. In these cases it is ok to treat other parts of the body such as the adrenals for shock.
- If you are Diabetic, Reiki can reduce the amount of insulin you need to have, so let your doctor monitor your dosage.
- Do not use Reiki to stomach, immediately after taking any medicine or else it will neutralize the effect.

POST TREATMENT CARE:

After treatment, mentally request Reiki to keep healing patient as long as he needs healing. Then, wash your hands thoroughly. You must do this even if you have not physically touched the patient.

This step is very necessary to remove the energy particles that have remained on your hand after the treatment. The reason for this is that these energy particles may be carrying the seeds of the ailment of the patient.

If you do not wash your hands immediately after healing, these particles may enter your body & produce the same symptoms for some time, & you may feel that you got the ailment of patient you healed.

When the treatment is over, after asking the patient how he feels, start the conversation about something totally different that is in no way connected with the ailment and healing. **Talk to the patient for some time, on this other subject.** This is *necessary to cut your connection from the patient after the healing session*.

If you do not do this, *there is a possibility that the patient may keep drawing the energy from you even later and as a result, you may feel depleted if you are not prepared for the energy transfer in this way.* These tips are necessary because those who do not follow them have a number of misconceptions about Reiki.

They feel that after you heal the patient, you get his ailment. After you heal all your energy is given to the patient and you feel weak. This does happen if the healer does not follow the above precautions. Of course this is not the fault of Reiki.

This happens because *along with Reiki energy, unknowingly, your own energy too gets involved in the healing. This energy is not as intelligent as Reiki. So you need to do this to cut this energy.*

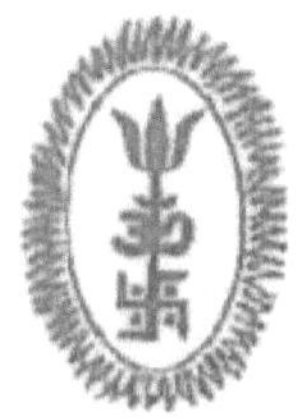

INTENTIONAL HEALING FOUNDATION

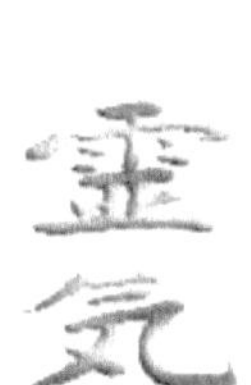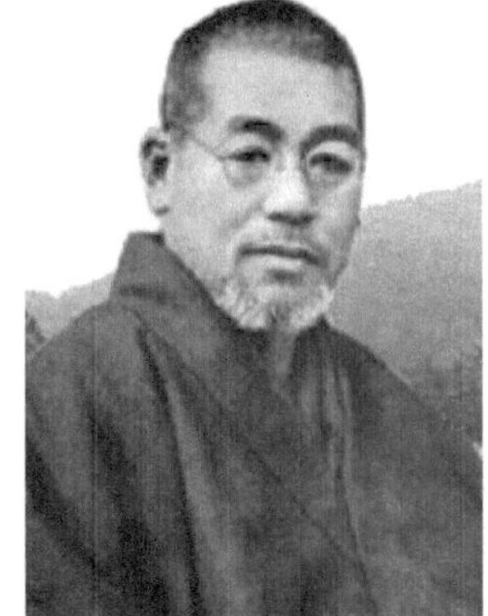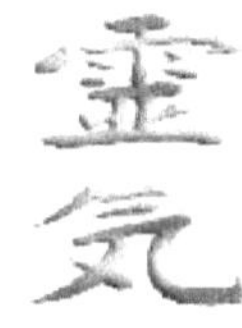

Reiki 2

CLASS LITERATURE

BY

DR. REKHAA KALE

9820044254 / 9870044254

rekhaa.kale@yahoo.com

REIKI-2

WHAT YOU LEARN IN REIKI-2

In Reiki-2 **Okuden** ("奥伝" in Japanese, meaning "Inner Teachings") one learns to heal events, distant things as well as patients who are at any far away distance, in absentee. Also one gets to know about symbols for healing.

In this level, one also learns about the original Sanskrit Mantras from which these symbols came. One learns how to use these symbols as well as mantras for more effective healing. One practices things like making an intention, writing an intention, visualizing the patient, visualizing event to be created or changed & so on. One practices the ways to heal a person from a distance for his whole body, as well as short form of healing method where he can heal just in ten minutes or so.

This means, by learning second level of Reiki, number of things one can work on is multiplied while time needed for healing is reduced. So, after learning the Reiki Symbols and their original Sanskrit Mantras, one learns of various possibilities in healing as well as creating future, one also learns different ways to use them.

After learning this, the student is attuned into Reiki 2. After attunement, he has to practice the healing once again. This lets him know the difference between feelings before and after attunement. Also seeker can get feedback from those whom he sends the healing before and after attunement. This feedback can help him know the difference the patient feels in the healing after the attunement of Reiki-2. Then the teacher gives some concluding tips and tells the student about the areas in life where he can use this healing method. These tips can be covering most of the areas, but still they cannot be exhaustive.

There are many areas in life where we can use Reiki. Your master need not know areas of your work, so he may leave out some areas in your life where you can use Reiki. It is you who have to locate and explore these areas. The teacher tells the student to experiment freely and use symbols & techniques in as many positive ways as he can. Normally, a master teacher also tells the student to practice regularly at least for 21 days. This is just to make sure that the student uses Reiki-2 well.

There are some who feel that one cannot learn the next degree before these 21 days. This is not so. One can learn the next degree any time when both you and your teacher feel that you are ready for the next level. Also a good Reiki teacher tells the student to feel free to ask for any support in the Reiki matter anytime he needs.

TRADITIONAL SYMBOLS

In traditional Reiki, we find three symbols. These are, HON SHA ZAI SHO NEN, SE HEI KI AND CHOKKOU REI. Let us see them in details:

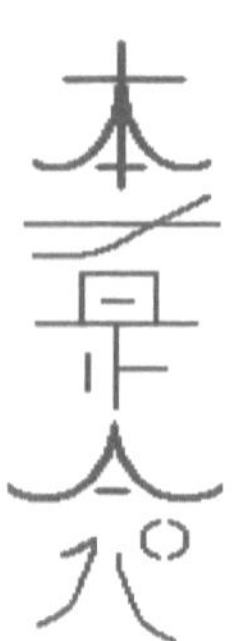

HON SHA ZAI SHO NEN is the bridge between the healer and the patient. In fact, it is a bridge between the event created by the healer in his mind, in his virtual reality, and the actual reality where that event must manifest. This has to be created before we start distance healing. As the healer draws this symbol, the knots of the karmas in the healer are released and the energies sent by the healer reach the patient freely.

The Buddhist chant from which this appears to have come is, **"HON SHA ZA SHA NEN"** "Oh lord, release all my Karmas!"

The Original Sanskrit Mantra that I found, from which this symbol appears to have originated is, **"HONG SAHA JOOM SAHA NAMAH"**. It means, "I invoke the creator, protector & destroyer (to heal) & request the protector to keep protecting." (Hong = Brahman, Saha = Vishnu, Joom = Mrityunjaya, Namah = salute)

The literal meaning of each part of this symbol is as follows:

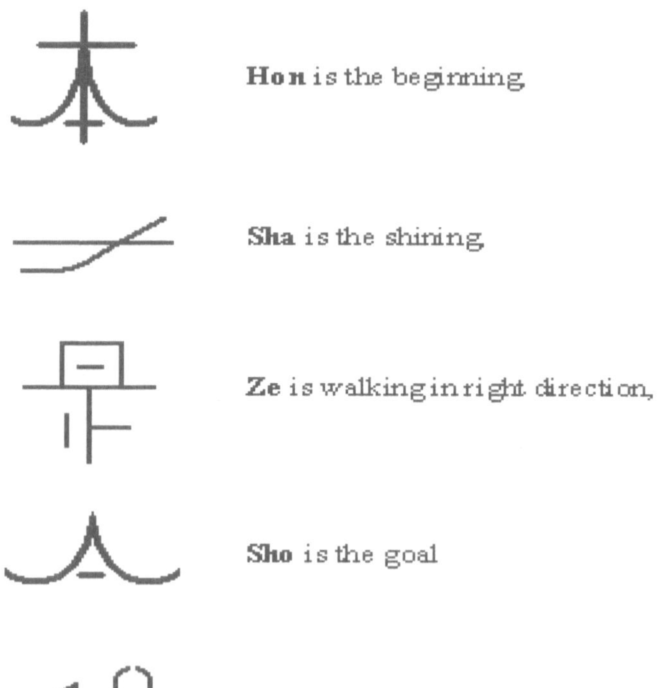

Hon is the beginning,

Sha is the shining,

Ze is walking in right direction,

Sho is the goal

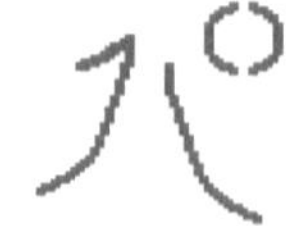

Nen is the opening in one's deepest being.

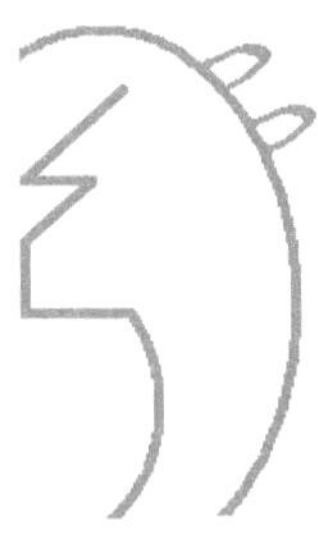

SE HEI KI is the symbol that clears the obstacles in the healing work. It also dissolves the physical, mental & emotional blocks in the healing. If there is any energy in disharmony, it also clears that disharmony.

The original Sanskrit Mantra that I found from which this might have originated is, "HASKLIM NAMAH". It means, *ha=earth, sa=water, ka=fire, la=air, ee=space, m=indicating plural*. So Haskleem namah means, "I salute & invoke earth, water, fire, air & space elements."

According to some, **SE HEI KI** has originated from the Sanskrit syllable, HRIH. The **HRIH** written in Sanskrit shows the similarity with **SE HEI KI** in its form.

The literal meaning of each part of this symbol is as follows:

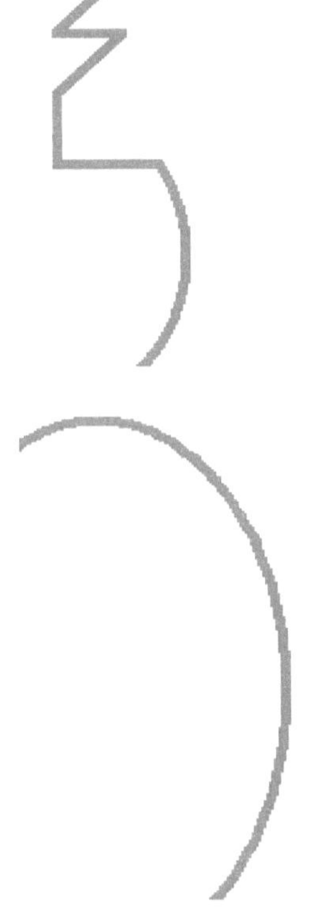

Se is invisible embryo source of external form.

He is the protecting force that dissolves all the wrong energies.

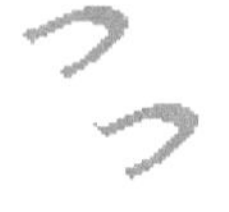

Ki is the life force energy.

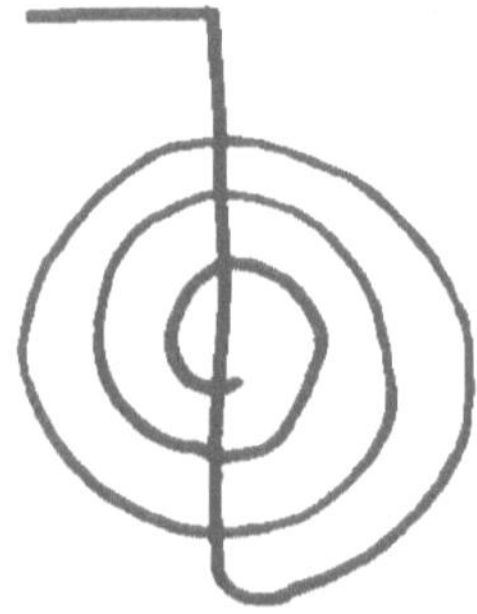

CHOKKOU REI is the symbol of power. This is used to empower the energy that is sent to a person, object or event. Whenever we are sending Reiki at a distance, to increase the speed of healing, we use this symbol. It is a catalyst that amplifies the projected energy.

The original Sanskrit word from which it is likely to have come is, **"CHAKRE"**. It means circular motion or spiralling movement. Here, one may even recite **"CHAM CHAKRAYA NAMAH"**, meaning, I invoke and salute the rotation of energy.

The literal meaning of each part of this symbol is as follows:

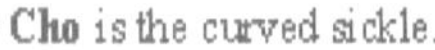 **Cho** is the curved sickle.

Ku is process of entering space to produce wholeness from where nothing exists.

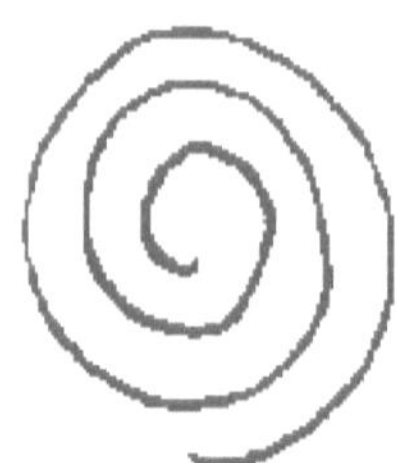 **Re** is universal, spiral essence of mystical power.

The order of drawing the symbols while giving Reiki is, *HON SHA ZAI SHO NEN, SE HEI KI & CHOKKOU REI.* Some follow just the reverse order. They draw CHOKKOU REI, SE HEI KI & HON SHA ZAI SHO NEN. Some draw CHOKKOU REI, HON SHA ZAI SHO NEN & SE HEI KI.

The logic that I have for using this order is, when you have to start distance healing, you must first have a path to travel. Without a path, you cannot go anywhere. Then you must remove all obstacles from it and then accelerate with your vehicle on it.

So, when we start any healing, the first thing we do is, create a path by drawing the path creator symbol, HON SHA ZAI SHO NEN. Then we draw the symbol that clears all the obstacles in the path of Reiki viz., SE HEI KI. Then we draw the symbol to speed up the Reiki sent viz., the power symbol, CHOKKOU REI.

The symbols HON SHA ZAI SHO NEN, SE HEI KI, as well as CHOKKOU REI are drawn with a number of variations. I am giving some of these variations. These are just for your reference. You can use only the variation you feel the best... All the variations are equally effective. The readers may use any of these variations.

69

Different Reiki teachers teach different variations. But actually the difference between them is as much as the difference between different fonts used in any language!

Please know that actually, there are just 3 symbols that are given above and the following are just different ways to write them.

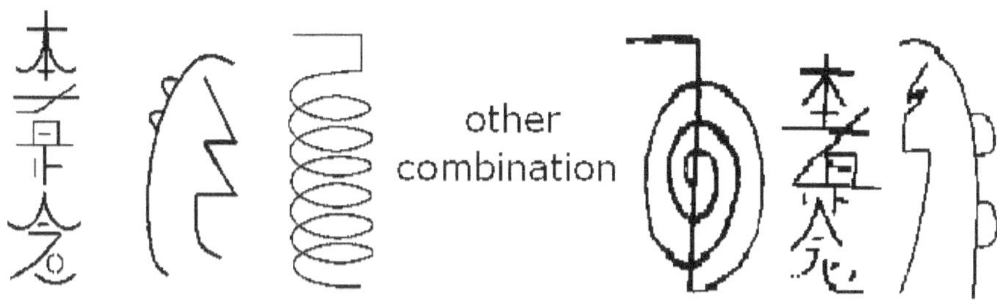

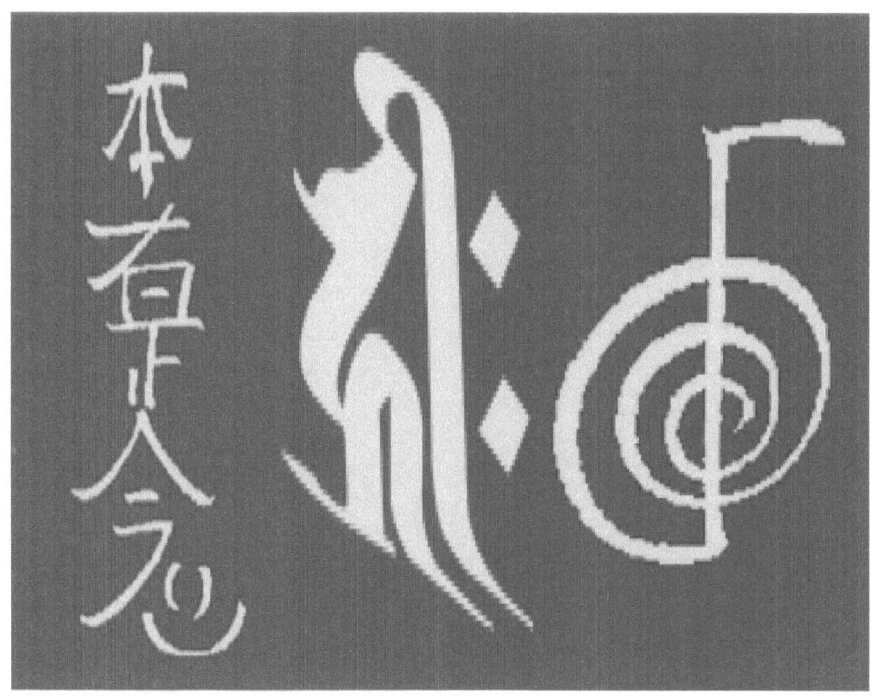

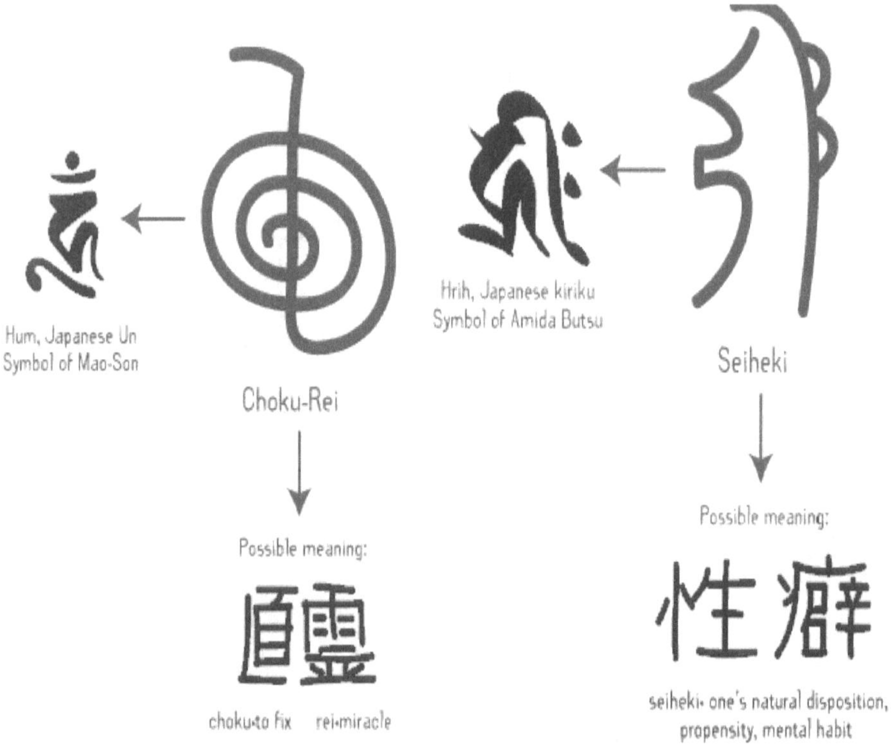
Hum, Japanese Un
Symbol of Mao-Son
Choku-Rei
Possible meaning:
直靈
choku-to fix
rei-miracle
Hrih, Japanese kiriku
Symbol of Amida Butsu
Seiheki
Possible meaning:
性癖
seiheki- one's natural disposition,
propensity, mental habit

Chokurei
Increase Power
Sei he Ki
Hon Sha Ze Sho Nen
absent Healing

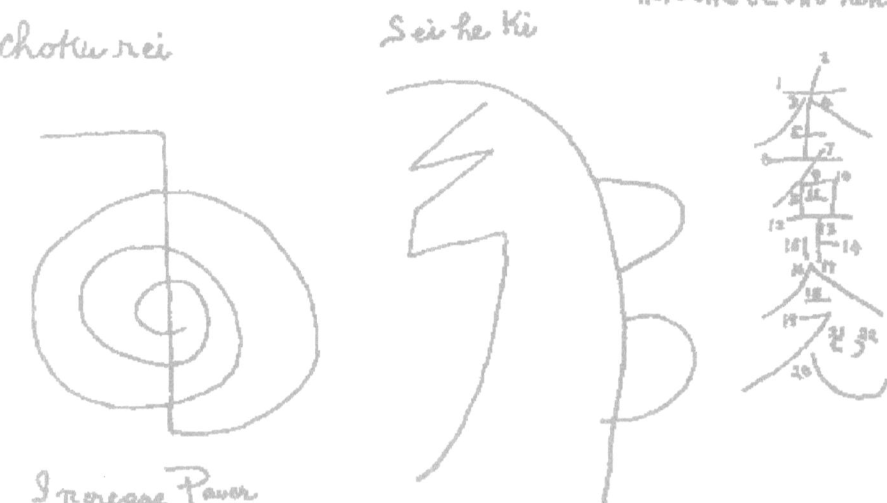

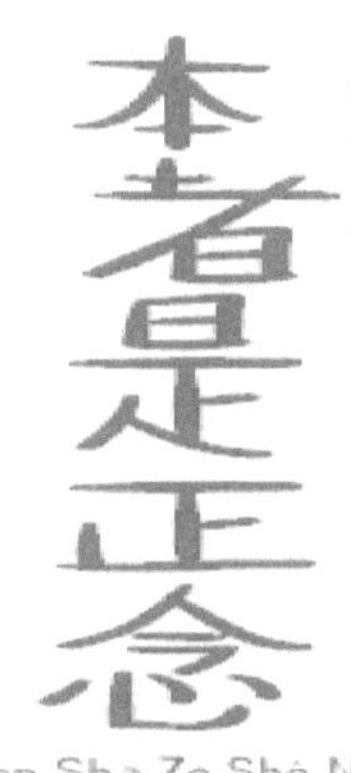

Hon Sha Ze Shō Nen
(full sentence)

Hon Sha Ze Shō Nen
(version I learned)

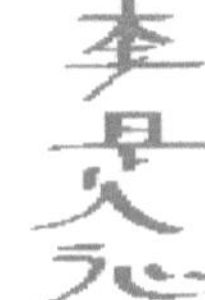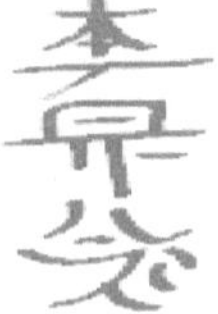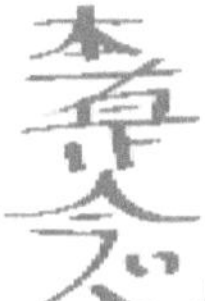

Other versions

Some Versions of HON SHA ZAI SHO NEN taught over the globe:

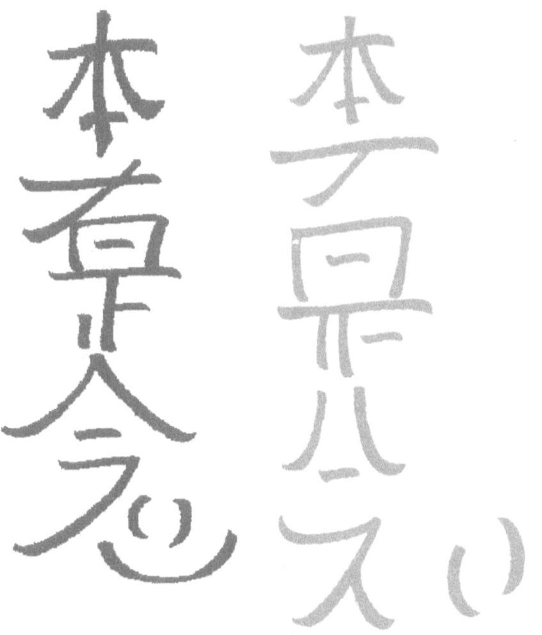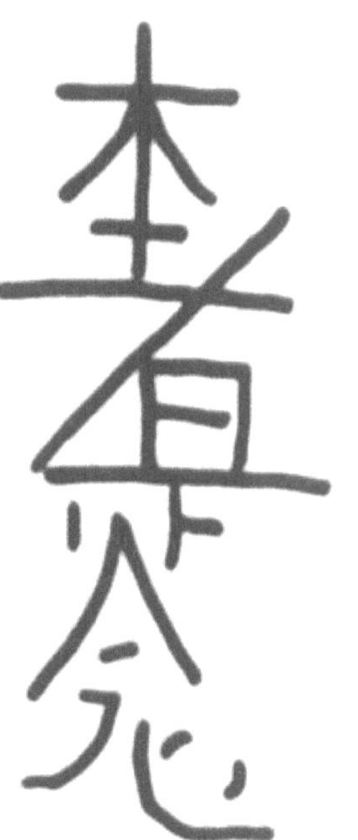

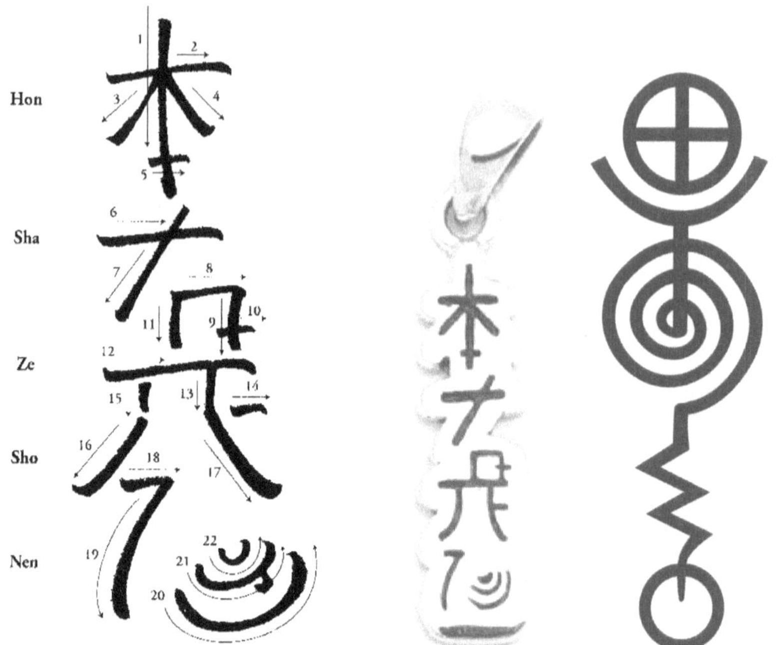

Hon
Sha
Ze
Sho
Nen

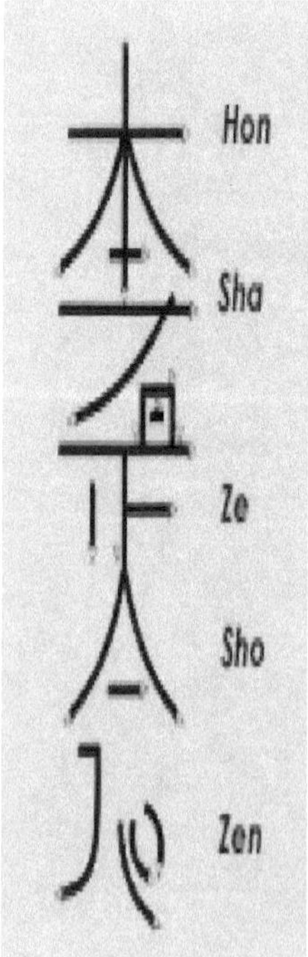

Hon
Sha
Ze
Sho
Zen

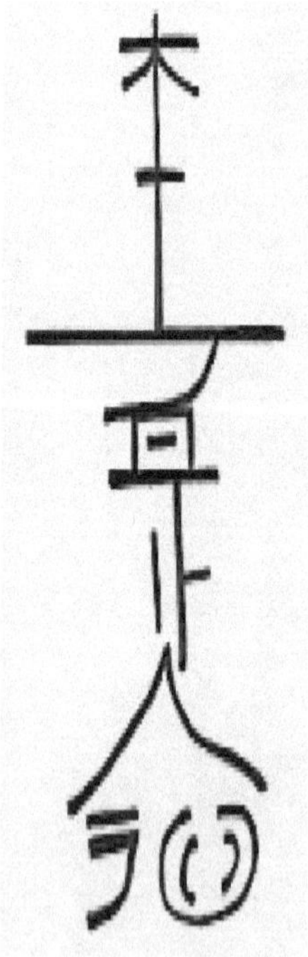

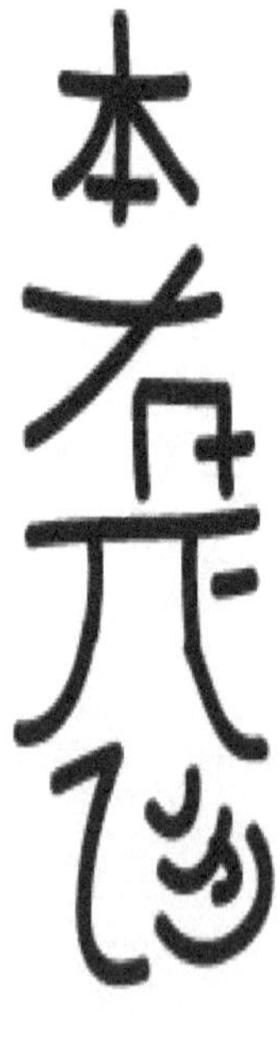

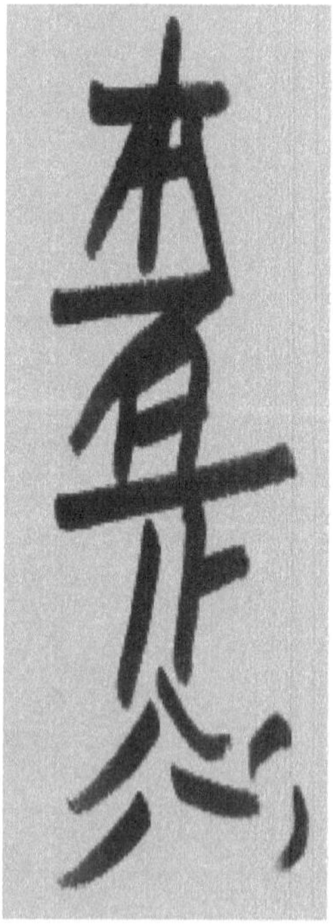

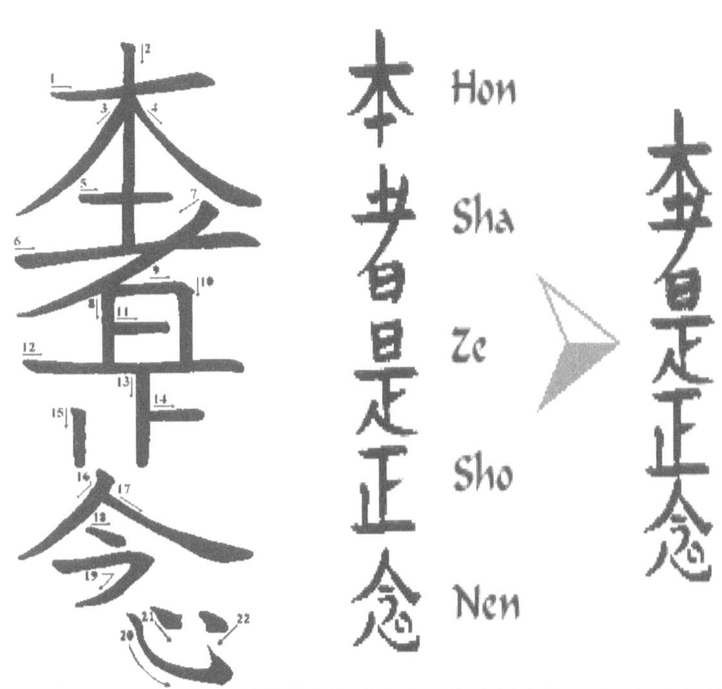

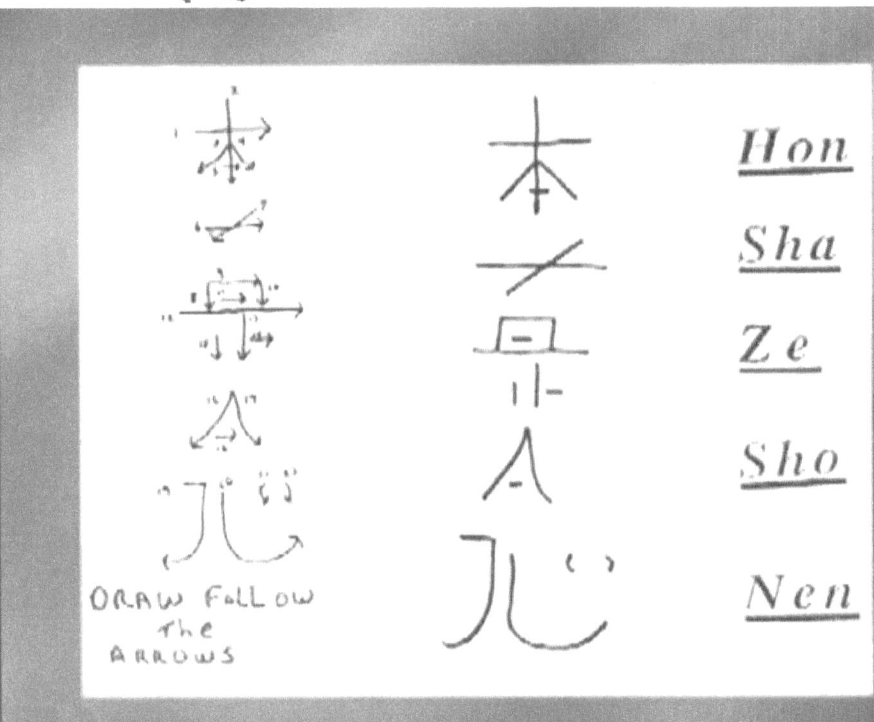

74

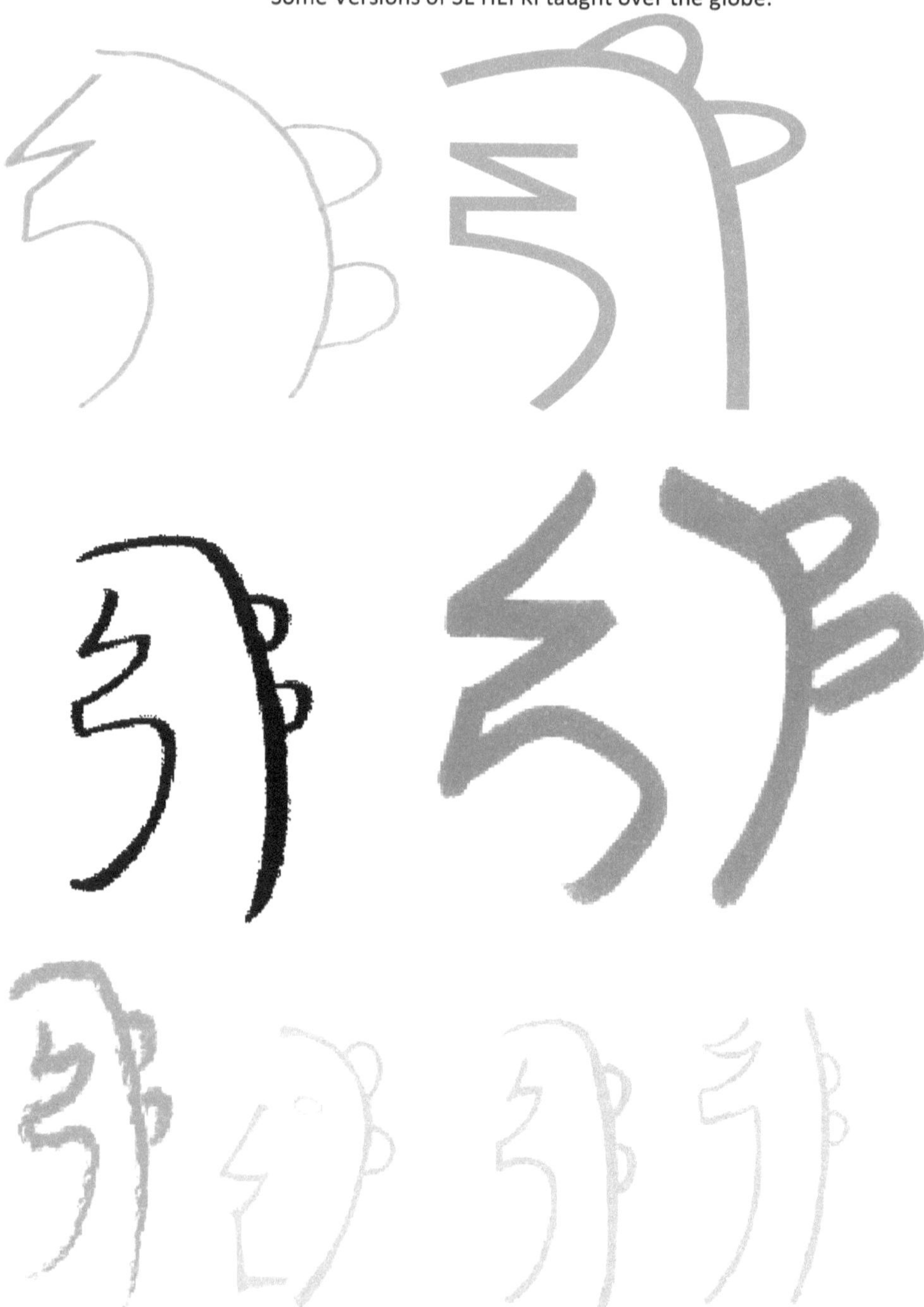

Some Versions of CHOKKOU REI taught over globe; for drawing with one hand as well as both hands:

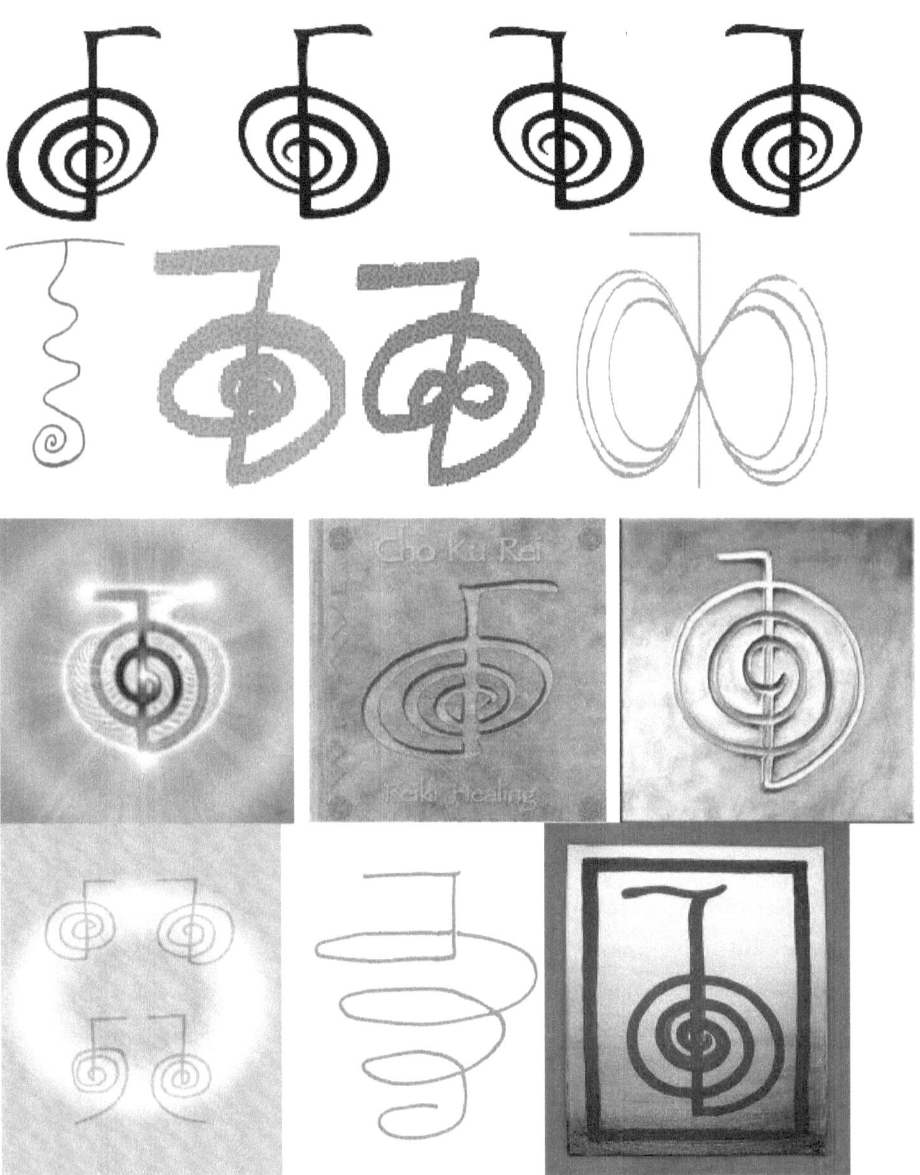

USE OF SYMBOLS

These symbols are used in different ways. Let us see them:

MAIN PROCEDURE FOR THE USE OF SYMBOLS:

@ **Visualize, see, imagine** or **declare** the *affected person, animal, area of the body, the object or the machine, the event you wish to create, thought you want to change, past thought, spirit you want to heal*. Or **write** the **intention** as if it has happened or materialised, on a paper. Put it in a **box**.

@ Make your vision as clear as possible. If you are visualizing or imagining, add as many details as you can to the image you visualize, so that the image will be almost complete as you want it to be.

@ (In common language, this is called ***covering*** the person, body part, animal, image or object ***with white light***)

@ Mentally draw three Reiki symbols over the visualized image.

@ Draw [symbol] Say **hon sha zai sho nen** 3 times

@ Draw [symbol] say **se hei ki** 3 times

@ Draw [symbol] say **chokkou rei** 3 times

@ Mentally give Reiki till you feel vibrations or heat.

@ Mentally draw symbols again over image with desired change.

@ Draw [symbol] Say **hon sha zai sho nen** 3 times

@ Draw [symbol] say **se hei ki** 3 times

@ Draw [symbol] say **chokkou rei** 3 times

@ Request Reiki to keep working till the event or thing needs energy to materialize the desired change and stop.

- Visualise as clearly as possible.

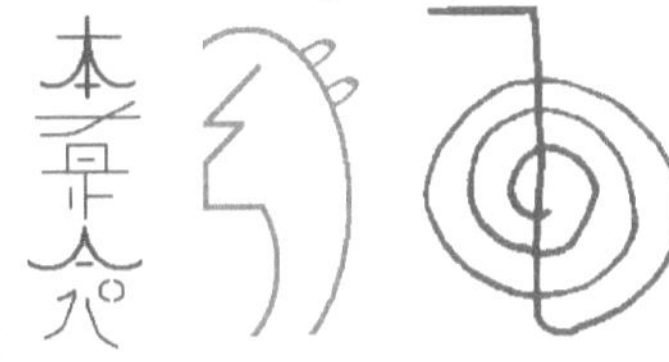

- Draw 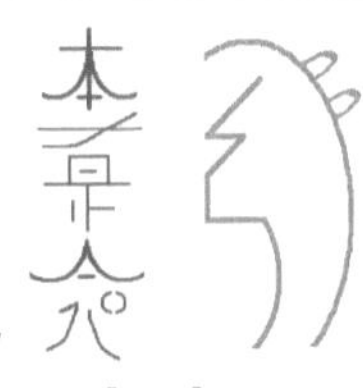 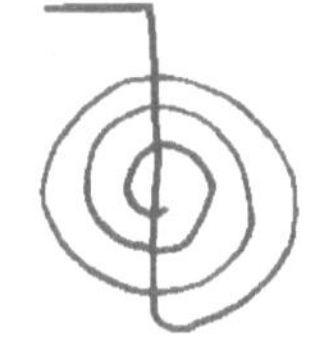 and say the names of each 3 times.
- Alternatively,
- Say **HONG SAHA JOOM SAHA NAMAH** 3 times
- Say HASKLIM NAMAH 3 times
- Say **CHAKRE** 3 times

Give Reiki for 5 to 10 minutes.

- Draw and say the names of each 3 times.
- Alternatively,
- Say **HONG SAHA JOOM SAHA NAMAH** 3 times
- Say HASKLIM NAMAH 3 times
- Say **CHAKRE** 3 times
- Stop.

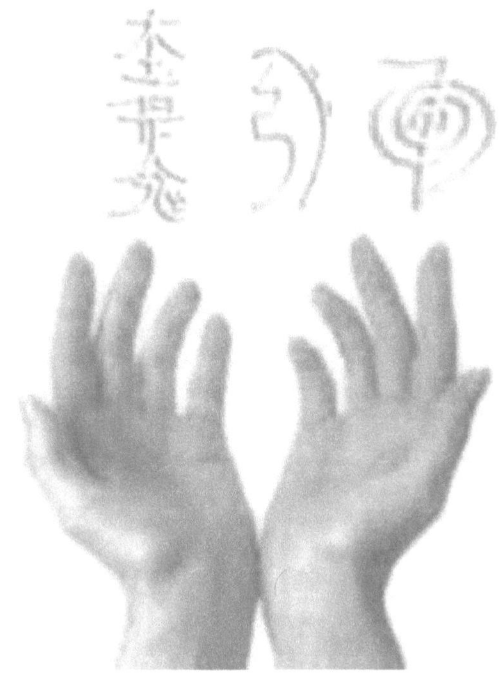

You may remember this as:

- Visualise
- Give Reiki
- Stop

Or

- Visualize
- Say **HONG SAHA JOOM SAHA NAMAH** 3 times
- Say **HASKLIM NAMAH** 3 times
- Say **CHAKRE** 3 times
- Reiki
- Say **HONG SAHA JOOM SAHA NAMAH** 3 times
- Say **HASKLIM NAMAH** 3 times
- Say **CHAKRE** 3 times
- Stop

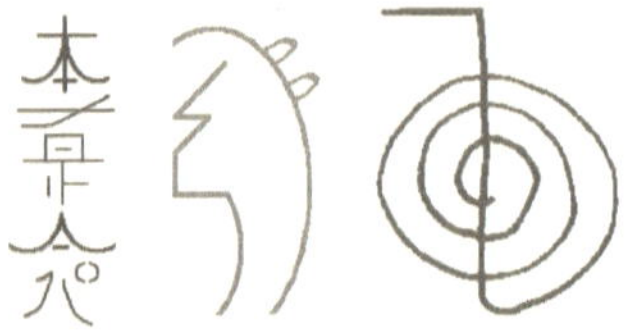

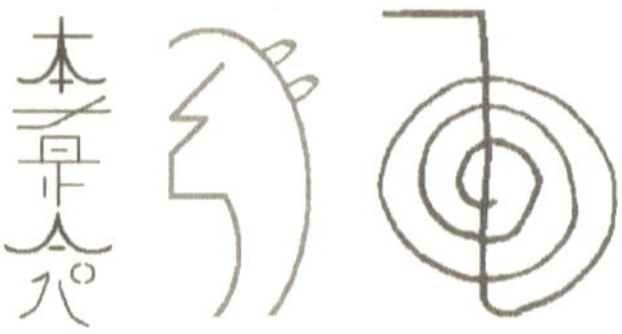

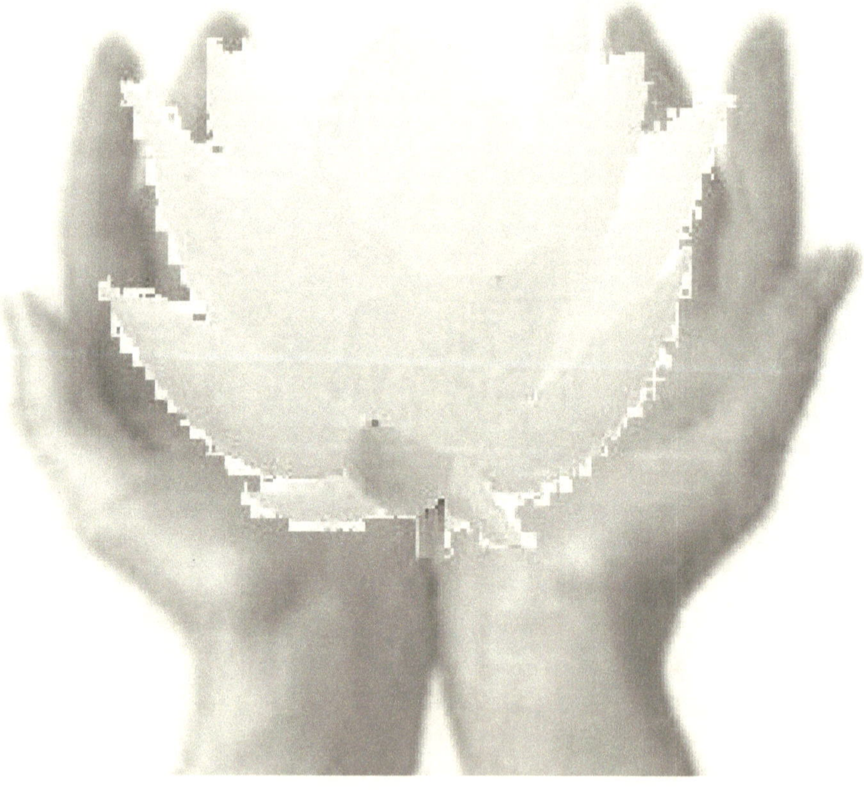

SHORT FORM OF ABSENTEE HEALING:

- Visualise the person or animal or plant you wish to heal.
- Make this image very clear.
- Imagine the person or animal or plant healed between your hands.

- Draw ⏚ Say **hon sha zai sho nen** 3 times

- Draw ⏚ say **se hei ki** 3 times

- Draw ⏚ say **chokkou rei** 3 times
- Visualize the person between the hands getting healed.
- Feel the energies going towards the object being healed.

- **Keep giving Reiki till the energy flow is felt.**
- When Reiki flow stops,

- Draw ⏚ Say **hon sha zai sho nen** 3 times

- Draw ⏚ say **se hei ki** 3 times

- Draw ⏚ say **chokkou rei** 3 times
- Stop.

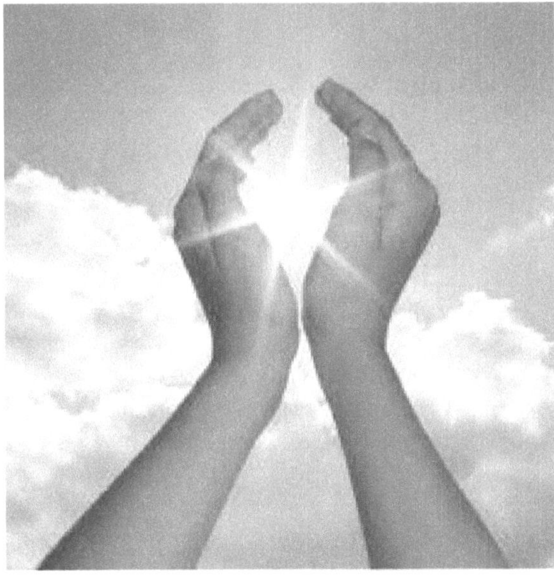

LONG FORM OF ABSENTEE HEALING:
(NOT ADVISED TO BE FOLLOWED UNLESS YOU ARE HEALING SOMEONE REALLY TOO CLOSE)

- Visualize the person to be healed.
- Visualise his problem.
- **Declare that your body is the body of the patient.**
- Declare that the Reiki is going to the patient.
- Give full self Reiki with symbols.

- Draw Say **hon sha zai sho nen** 3 times

- Draw say **se hei ki** 3 times

- Draw say **chokkou rei** 3 times

- **Every time, mentally declare that patient is healed.**

- **Give special attention on the points with problem.**

- **Place the hands on them till the Reiki is passing.**

- When you finish, thank Reiki for healing the patient.

- Draw Say **hon sha zai sho nen** 3 times

- Draw say **se hei ki** 3 times

- Draw say **chokkou rei** 3 times

- **Declare that your body now is yours and stop.**

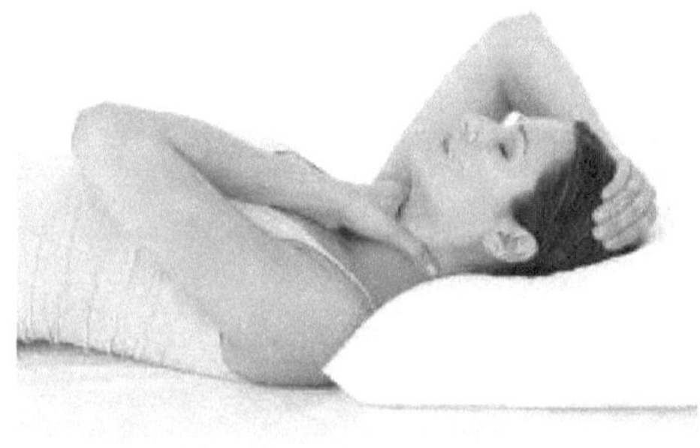

CREATING THE FUTURE:

- @ Visualise the event that you want to create with all possible details.
- @ Visualise the date and time desired for the event to happen.

- @ Draw Say **hon sha zai sho nen** 3 times

- @ Draw say **se hei ki** 3 times

- @ Draw say **chokkou rei** 3 times

- @ **Give Reiki for 5 to 10 minutes.**

- @ Draw Say **hon sha zai sho nen** 3 times

- @ Draw say **se hei ki** 3 times

- @ Draw say **chokkou rei** 3 times

- @ (Repeat the process till the event is created in reality)

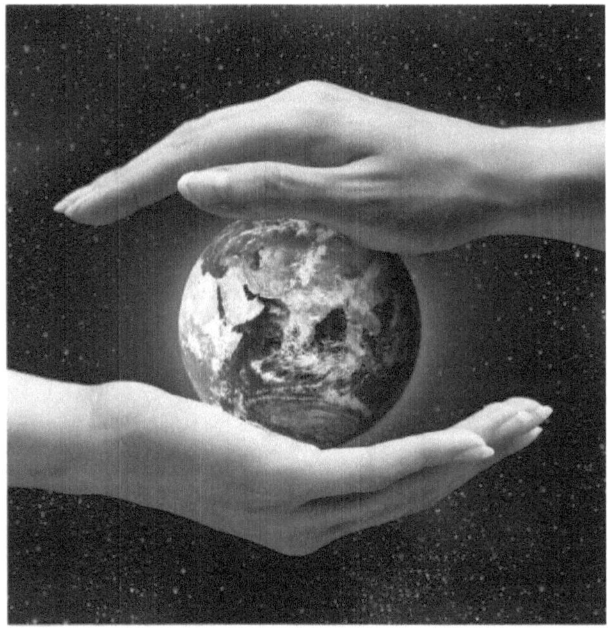

REIKI BOX:

- Write intention on paper as you would, after completion.
- Let your intention be like; _____________ (patient's full name) is totally healed of _____________.
- Hold the paper in your hands.
- You can write many intentions this way.
- Put them into a box.
- Hold the box in hands.
- Cover it with white light.
- Draw ⧖ Say **hon sha zai sho nen** 3 times

- Draw ⧖ say **se hei ki** 3 times

- Draw ◎ say **chokkou rei** 3 times

- **Give Reiki for 5 to 10 minutes.**

- Draw ⧖ Say **hon sha zai sho nen** 3 times

- Draw ⧖ say **se hei ki** 3 times

- Draw ◎ say **chokkou rei** 3 times
- Keep the paper / box in a proper place and stop.
- (Do this twice a day till the intension is completed.)

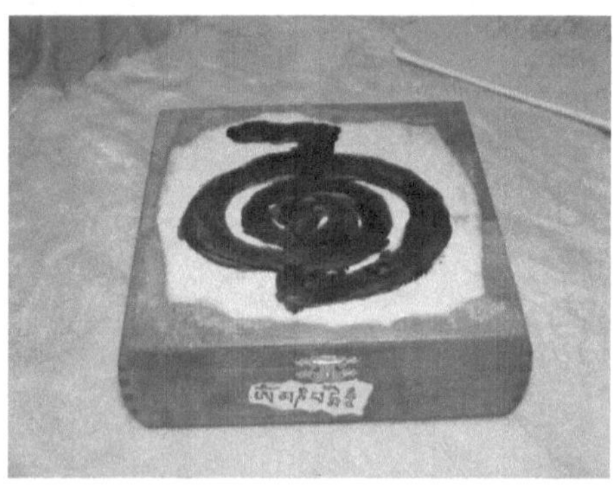

MENTAL METHOD OF HEALING:

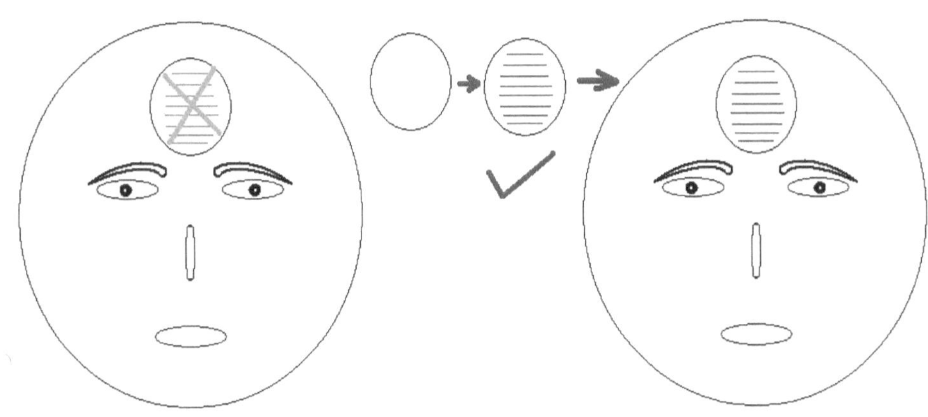

@ See the third eye of the person opening.

@ *Erase* the *negative* thoughts in it.
@ *Write* the *desired positive* thought in it thrice.

@ Draw Say **hon sha zai sho nen** 3 times

@ Draw say **se hei ki** 3 times

@ Draw say **chokkou rei** 3 times

@ **Give Reiki for 5 to 10 minutes.**

@ Draw Say **hon sha zai sho nen** 3 times

@ Draw say **se hei ki** 3 times

@ Draw say **chokkou rei** 3 times
@ Close the third eye.

AURA LOOSENING:

- Make a person sit / lie down in a comfortable position.
- Move your hands around 2 to 3 inches away from the body.
- Feel the blocks if any, and remove them physically.
- Make the Aura loose in general, with your hands.
- Feel the patient becoming free from depression, & tensions.
- Cover the patient with white light.

- Draw ⟨symbol⟩ Say **hon sha zai sho nen** 3 times

- Draw ⟨symbol⟩ say **se hei ki** 3 times

- Draw ⟨symbol⟩ say **chokkou rei** 3 times

- **Give Reiki for 5 to 10 minutes.**

- Draw ⟨symbol⟩ Say **hon sha zai sho nen** 3 times

- Draw ⟨symbol⟩ say **se hei ki** 3 times

- Draw ⟨symbol⟩ say **chokkou rei** 3 times
- **Draw Golden Se hei ki, on all the six sides of person.**
-

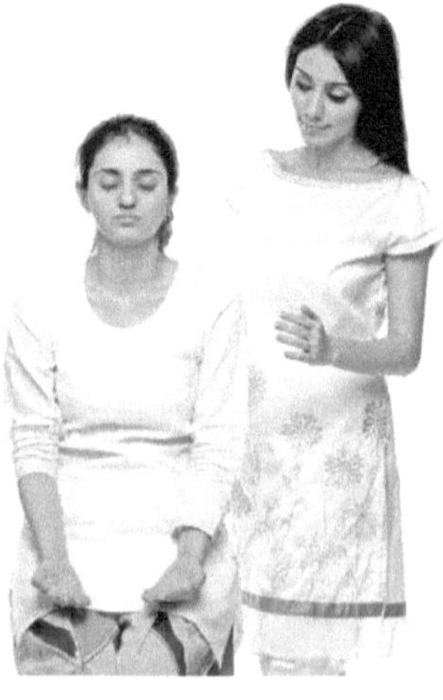

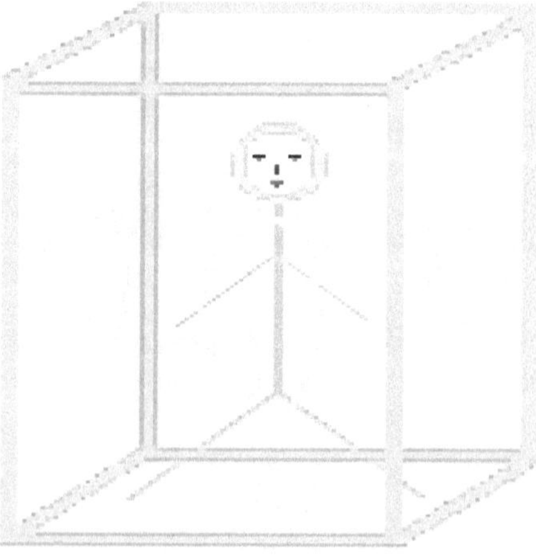

Methods taught by others but omitted by me:

There are a few methods that many teachers teach in Reiki 2, but I have omitted them as I have found them either illogical or erroneous. I also found that in some of these methods, one may have adverse effects, energy infections or psychological problems due to excessive use of these methods.

HEALING THE DEAD

1. Imagine the dead person
2. Visualise him as alive and getting up
3. Visualise you completing the unfinished communication with him/her.
4. Visualise the person (who is actually dead now) to be happy
5. Now visualise the person dead again
6. Give Reiki to whole event.

HEALING THE PAST

1. Imagine the past unwanted event
2. Visualise it changing as you wanted it to be
3. Visualise you happy in the desired situation.
4. Visualise people in past around as you wanted them to be
5. Now visualise the present again
6. Give Reiki to whole event.

HEALING THE CHILDHOOD

1. Imagine the past unwanted event in childhood
2. Visualise it changing as you wanted it to be
3. Visualise you as happy child in the desired situation.
4. Visualise people in past around as you wanted them to be
5. Now visualise the present again
6. Give Reiki to yourself as a child in past.

HEALING THE RELATIONSHIP
(BETWEEN TWO UNKNOWN PEOPLE)

1. Imagine two persons with bad relations
2. Visualise them as friends and hugging each other
3. Visualise them having great relation with each other
4. Visualise persons(who are actually enemies) to be happy together
5. Now Give Reiki to both persons and the imagined picture.

HEALING TREES

1. Hold a tree or plant between your hands
2. Give Reiki to it for 10 minutes
3. Do this every day and tree will grow well

HEALING THE HOUSE

1. Place your hands on each wall of your house.
2. Give Reiki to each wall.
3. Declare that the house is healed.
4. Do this daily.

HEALING THE CAR

1. Place your hands on the car bonnet.
2. Give Reiki to it for 10 minutes.
3. Declare that the car is healed.
4. You will find that car is giving higher mileage.
5. Do this daily.

HEALING THE FINANCES

1. Hold your wallet in hands.
2. Wish that it stays full.
3. Give Reiki to it for 10 minutes
4. Keep it back in pocket
5. You will get lot of money.

REIKI OPERATION

1. Imagine the person to be healed
2. Imagine the affected body area of the patient.
3. Mentally cut the aura of that area.
4. Mentally remove the bad energies from it.
5. Mentally stitch the aura.
6. Mentally apply healing lotion on the stitched area.
7. Declare the patient to be healed.

The above methods are some of the ones that are taught even today by many Reiki teachers but make no sense to any logical minded person. So I have omitted them.

CHAKRAS

Charkas are the energy centres through which we breathe in the energy in our body. These are very small perforations in the body that cannot be even seen with normal eye. When we see the aura, we find that near this area, the energy around the body becomes like a funnel. The area where we find this funnel like structure, we find the energy rotating clockwise or anti-clockwise. It is due to these rotations that these energy centres are known as charkas i.e. the rotating circles. Very few actually know about this real nature of charkas. Generally people talk things stated about charkas in some books without understanding or feeling the charkas at all! Such people show that they know something great as they talk about charkas or other things of spirituality. In fact they have only hearsay knowledge!

Charkas are the entry and exit points of plasma or the life force energy as well as any other energy in the body. These are very minute openings that are just not visible with eyes or even with microscope! The energies enter the body or leave the body thro' these points. The chakra (the Sanskrit word for wheel) is the energy centres or vortex in your aura that governs & regulates the energy entering & flowing throughout the physical & energy bodies. They are energy structures not physical organs. The chakras are aligned along the central channel which runs along the spinal cord.

Energies move up and down and also in a spiral in and out along this channel and side channels called Ida and Pingala. The Caduceus, an ancient symbol of the Healing arts is said to represent this flow.

There are many chakras major and minor. In fact each joint of the body contains a chakra. The inner side of the joint has the front portion of the chakra and the outer position has the back position of the chakra. But the seven major chakras are the ones that control the whole system. These are: - 1: Root, 2: sacral (Mid stomach), 3: Solar plexus, 4: Heart, 5: Throat, 6: Brow & 7: Crown,

The Reiki hand positions cover the main chakra centres and the main meridian channels that the life force flows through. Running energy into the feet will facilitate energy flow through all the major channels. This is the reason why we have the primary information of the chakras while learning Reiki. In the advance levels of Reiki, if we cannot give the full body Reiki, healing the chakras also works to produce total general healing!

DETAILED INFORMATION OF CHAKRAS:

@ Root Chakra: Muladhara is a Seat of KUNDALINI. It is RED- black and is located at the perineum under the tail bone at the base of spine. Element that governs this chakra is earth + mineral kingdom. The sense controlled by this chakra is smell. The note of this chakra is c. The mantra of it is lam or e as in red. Its vortex or petals are 4. It governs Physical Awareness, vigour, heredity, survival, security, passion, feet, legs, survival, trust, home, money & job relation.

@ Sacral Chakra: Swadhisthana is a Seat of self. It is ORANGE, brown and is located at the sex organs or near belly button. Element that governs this chakra is water+ plant kingdom. The sense controlled by this chakra is taste. The note of this chakra is d. The mantra of it is vam or o as in home: vortex or petals 6. It governs anger, fear, social awareness, sexuality, creativity, emotions, nurturing, spleen, food or sex perceptions.

@ is a seat of power. It is YELLOW and is located between the sternum bone and the belly. Element that governs this chakra is fire+ animal kingdom. The sense controlled by this chakra is sight. The note of this chakra is d. The mantra of it is ram or Aum. Its vortex or petals are 10. It governs Intellectual Awareness, power, accomplishments, will, ego projections, vital energy control, freedom to be oneself.

@ Heart Chakra: Anahat is a Seat of love. It is GREEN, pink and is located at the heart in centre of chest. Element that governs this chakra is air+ human kingdom. The sense controlled by this chakra is touch. The note of this chakra is f#. The mantra of it is yam or a as in ah. Its vortex or petals are 12. It governs Emotional and Security Awareness, love, compassion, mediates between higher and lower planes of being healing, lungs, breath, Prana, sense of time, relationships in life.

@ Throat Chakra: Vishuddha is a Seat of creativity. It is SKY BLUE and is located at the base of throat. Element that governs this chakra is ether+ angelic realms. The sense controlled by this chakra is hearing. The note of this chakra is g#. The mantra of it is ham or u as in blue. Its vortex or petals are 16. It governs speech, voice, listening, hearing, total self expression, communication, conceptual awareness & ideas.

@ Third Eye Chakra: Ajna is a Seat of intuition. It is INDIGO and is located in the centre of forehead above eyes. Element that governs this chakra is spiritual+ vision of archangels. The sense controlled by this chakra is telepathy. The note of this chakra is high a. The mantra of it is Aum, OM or mmm. Its vortex or petals are 96. It governs Intuitive Awareness, intuition, thought, imagination, association of experiences, inner & outer sight, visions, memory, assimilation of perception, dreams.

@ Crown Chakra: Sahastrara is a Seat of the spirit. It is VIOLET, white and is located at the top of head. Element that governs this chakra is cosmic kingdom. Its mantra is Aum, ee as in bee. Its vortex or petals are 972. It governs imaginative awareness, connection to cosmic consciousness, spiritual wisdom, desires, true knowledge.

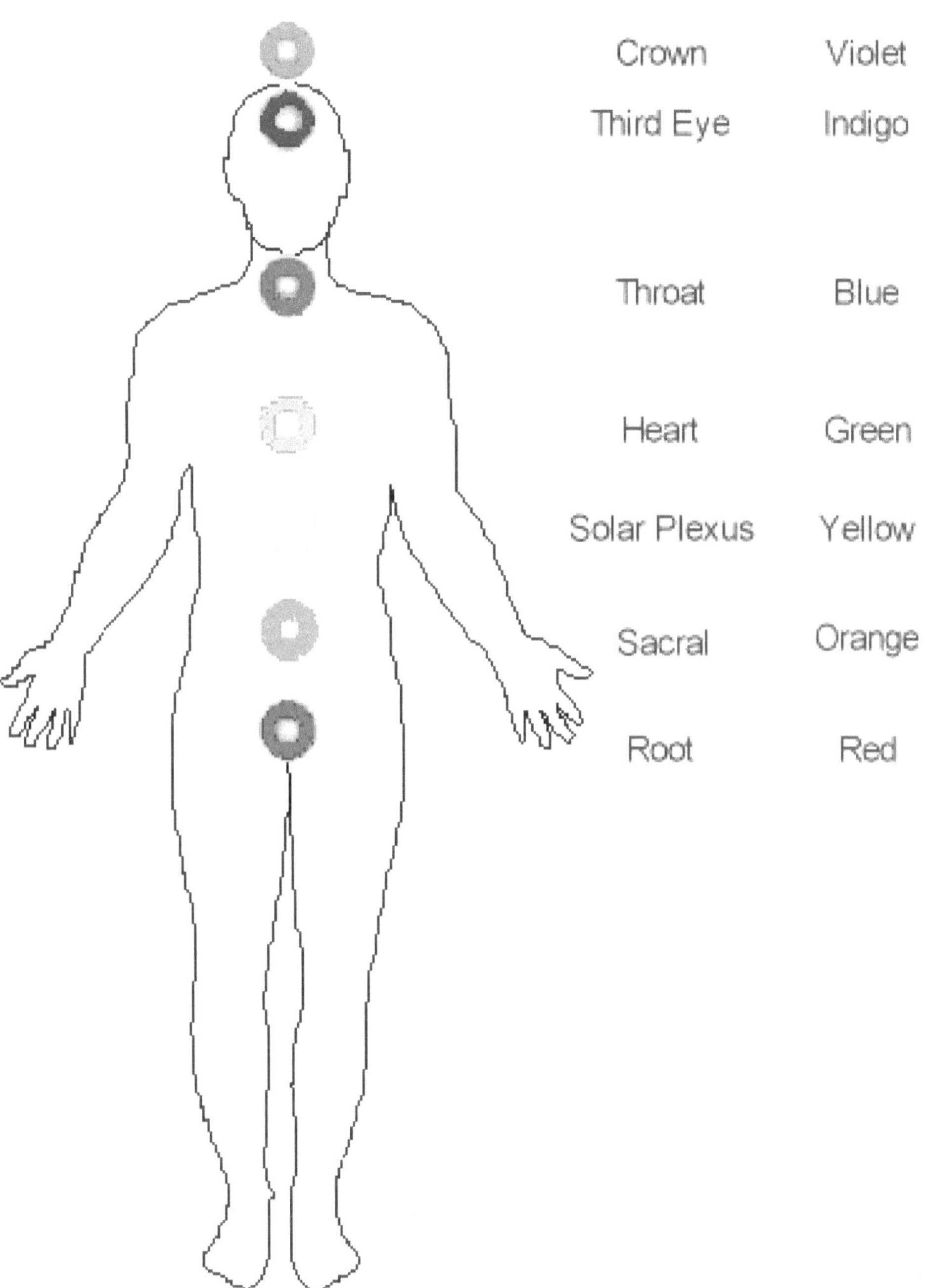

Crown	Violet
Third Eye	Indigo
Throat	Blue
Heart	Green
Solar Plexus	Yellow
Sacral	Orange
Root	Red

	ROOT	HARA	HEART	THROAT	THIRD EYE	CROWN
NAME	MOOLADHARA	SWADHISTHANA		VISHUDDHA	AJNA	SAHASTRARA
COLOUR	RED	ORANGE		TURQUOISE	INDIGO	VIOLET
PETALS	4	6		16	96	972
ELEMENT	EARTH	WATER		SPACE	SPACE	SPACE
SOUND	LAM	VAM		HAM	AUM	EEM
SENSE	SMELL	TASTE		HEARING	ESP	EMPATHY
GLAND	ADRENALS	GONADS		THYROID	PITUITARY	PINEAL
SYSTEM	BONES, LYMPH, EXCRETION	REPRODUCTIVE ASSIMILATION		GROWTH METABOLISM	ENDOCRINE	NERVOUS
NERVES	SACRAL PLEXUS	LUMBER PLEXUS		CERVICAL PLEXUS	CAROTID PLEXUS	BRAIN
AREA OF KNOWING	SAFETY, MONEY, TRUST, SURVIVAL, HOME, JOB, SECURITY	SENSATIONS, EMOTIONS, FEELINGS, FOOD, SEX, HUNGER		EXPRESSION, RECEPTION, ABUNDANCE, FLOWING, MANIFESTATION, LISTENING TO INTUITION	SPIRITUAL AWARENESS, PERSONAL AWARENESS, INSTINCT KNOWLEDGE	UNITY, UNIVERSAL AWARENESS, SOURCE OF INTUITION
ACTUAL POSITION IN BODY	PERINEUM POINT BETWEEN ANAL/URINARY OPENINGS	TWO FINGERS BELOW NAVAL BUTTON		LOWER HOLLOW PART OF FRONT NECK	CENTRE OF HEAD	TOP OF HEAD
BODY PART CONNECTED	KIDNEYS, BLADDER & SPINE	REPRODUCTIVE ORGANS		THROAT & LUNGS	HYPOTHALAMUS & TOTAL AUTONOMOUS NERVOUS SYSTEM	UPPER BRAIN & RIGHT EYE
FUNCTION CONTROLS	WATER & PHOSPHORUS CONTENT, CREATION OF SEX HORMONES.	APAN VAYU ALL PARTS BELOW DIAPHRAGM, MOVEMENT OF STOOLS & URINE.		AIR, LUNGS, HEART, TEMPERATURE, CALCIUM LEVEL, ENERGY PRODUCTION	AIR & SPACE, BODY GROWTH, BRAIN POWER, MEMORY	WATER BALANCE, WORKING OF GLANDS, CEREBRO-SPINAL FLUID, SEX DESIRE, NERVE-GROWTH

HOW TO MENTALLY CREATE AN EVENT:

- To create an event mentally,
- First of all remove all doubts from your mind about the event.
- Then, imagine it as you want it to happen.
- Try to see as many details as you can.
- Keep visualizing the event as you draw symbols over it.
- See the event more clearly as you close the symbols and stop.
- Stop thinking of the event after you stop giving Reiki.

PROCESS TO VISUALISE, IMAGINE OR DECLARE:

- Think of the event that you want to create
- Think of the details you want in it.
- Think how it will look when it manifests.
- Mentally create a scene where this event is happening.
- Keep seeing this scene as you see a movie.
- Try to create a mental picture, and if not, mentally declare that this event is happening.
- As you keep seeing this scene, you may see some problems in its materialising too.
- Think how those problems can go away and create a scene where these problems are not there.
- Once you are satisfied with the scene you have mentally created, take it as the event you want to work on with Reiki.

HOW TO WRITE A CORRECT INTENTION:

- To write a correct intention, remember the following:
- Write the intention as clearly as possible.
- Write the intention as briefly as possible.
- Write the intention as affirmatively as possible.
- Write the intention as you would write after it is completed.
- If possible, put even the date and time when you want the intention to happen.

Check the intentions you had written or imagined earlier applying these rules & correct them.

IDEAL MEDITATION FOR REIKI 2 HEALERS:

BALANCING OF CHAKRAS

- Sit in a comfortable position.
- Close your eyes.
- Feel your crown and root charkas.
- Allow the divine energies flow thro' them.
- Feel the energies in them getting balanced.
- Feel your third eye and sacral charkas.
- Allow the divine energies flow thro' them.
- Feel the energies in them getting balanced.
- Feel your throat and solar plexus charkas.
- Allow the divine energies flow thro' them.
- Feel the energies in them getting balanced.
- Feel the alignment of all these charkas.
- Feel your heart charka.
- Allow the divine energies flow thro' it.
- Feel the energies in it getting balanced.
- Feel your heart in alignment with other charkas.
- Feel the energies of all the charkas vibrating.
- Slowly open your eyes and start the routine.

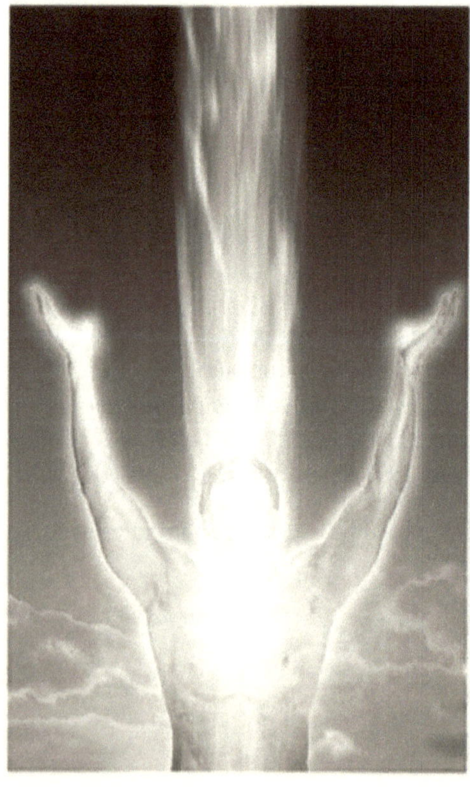

WORKING ON INTENTIONS AND BLOCKS:

1: Find out and list out the things that you want to heal in your life.
2: Write down these wishes as you would write them after they are completed.
3: Imagine your desires as if you are seeing them as fulfilled.

Do these exercises for at least 10 desires in your life.
Locate the thoughts that are stopping you from having the desires fulfilled.
Draw the symbols as you draw while giving Reiki.
Give Reiki to your naval.
Have an intention to release all blocking thoughts for 10 minutes.
Feel that all mental, emotional and spiritual blocks are getting released.
Feel confident that now no thought of yours will block your desires.
Draw the symbols as you draw while closing Reiki.
Stop.

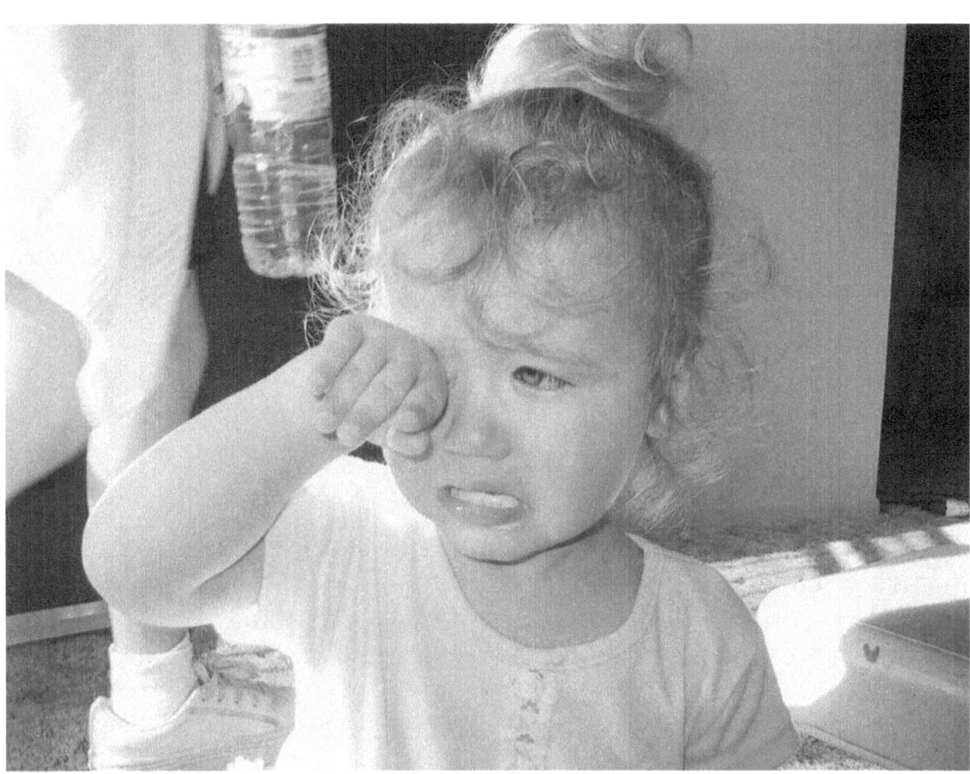

ACTIVATING WATER WITH REIKI:

To heal faster, and to heal the persons whose ailment you cannot diagnose, you can use the water activated with Reiki. To activate water with Reiki, you can do the following:

@ Take a glass full of water.

@ Think of the person to be healed.

@ Mentally request Reiki to create medicine needed for that person in the water in your hand.

@ Cover the glass of water with your hands, one hand over the water covering the glass and other below the glass.

@ Mentally start chanting **"HONG SAHA JOOM SAHA NAMAH"**

@ Say this for about 10 minutes.

@ Now chant the second mantra; **"HASKLIM NAMAH"**

@ Say this for about 5 minutes.

@ Now chant the third mantra; **"CHAKRE"**

@ Say this for about 2 minutes.

@ Once you have done this, the power of mantras will change the taste of water, creating the necessary medicine for patient in water.

@ Now that glass of water will have the capacity to heal the patient.

@ Give that glass of water to the patient you wish to heal.

@ Let the person drink that water completely at one time.

@ Now watch the patient getting healed.

You can do this daily for 21 days or more in case of a patient in case of chronic ailments.

Also, you can do it for yourself for your regular healing if you do not have much time to heal yourself with regular healing methods.

This is a shortest and most effective way to use Reiki 2.

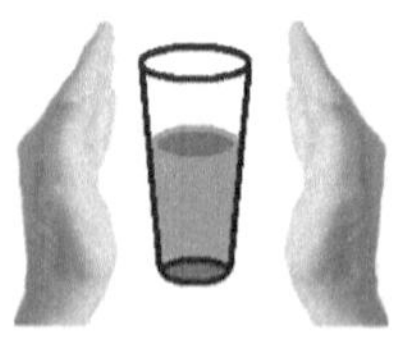

THINGS YOU CAN WORK ON WITH REIKI 2:

- ALL TYPES OF EVENTS
- SPIRITUAL GROWTH
- RELATIONSHIPS
- ENVIRONMENT
- THOUGHTS
- STABILITY
- FINANCES
- ENERGIES
- WEATHER
- ANIMALS
- MEMORY
- HABITS
- NATURE
- HEALTH
- THINGS
- PLANTS
- PLACES
- FUTURE
- PAST
- EGO
- ANY OTHER THINGS YOU CAN THINK OF...

BENEFITS OF REIKI 3 OVER REIKI 2
= WHY IS IT ADVISABLE NOT TO STOP REIKI QUEST AT REIKI 2?

- REIKI 2 HELPS US TO HEAL DISTANT THINGS.

- IT OPENS THE PENDORAS BOX OF CREATIVITY.

- BUT REIKI 3 TEACHES US HOW TO USE THIS.

- WITH REIKI 3, WE CAN DETECT THE PROBLEM.

- WE CAN FIND THE ROOT CAUSE OF PROBLEM.

- THEN WE WORK DIRECTLY ON THE ROOT.

- THIS NOT ONLY HELPS US HEAL FASTER, BUT ALSO HELPS US TO HEAL MORE EFFECTIVELY WITHOUT A POSSIBILITY OF RELAPSE OF ANY PROBLEM.

- STOPPING AT REIKI 2 IS LIKE ACQUIRING SOME ABILITY, BUT NOT WISHING TO USE IT TO ITS FULLEST.

- WHEN WE LEARN TO HEAL AT REIKI 2 LEVEL, WE GET THE ABILITY TO TRANSMIT HEALING ENERGY ANYWHERE, BUT REIKI 3 GIVES US THE ABILITY TO DETECT THE ACTUAL PROBLEM AND DO A PERFECT DIAGNOSIS THAT CAN ALWAYS BE CROSS CHECKED WITH REPORTS OF MEDICAL TESTS.

- SUCH AN ACCURATE DIAGNOSIS MAKER A HEALER PERFECT.

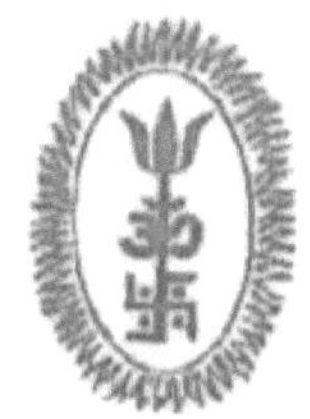

INTENTIONAL HEALING FOUNDATION

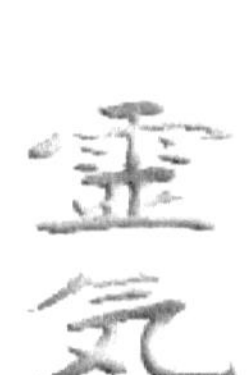
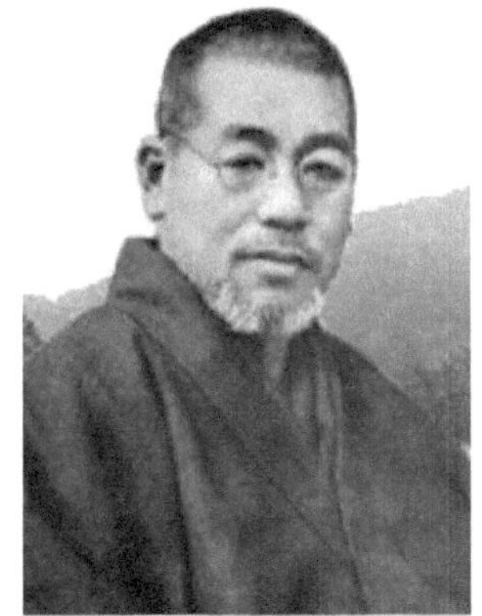
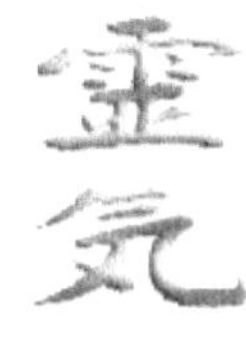

Reiki 3

CLASS LITERATURE

BY

DR. REKHAA KALE

9820044254 / 9870044254

rekhaa.kale@yahoo.com

REIKI-3

WHAT YOU LEARN IN REIKI-3

In Reiki-3 **Shinpiden** ("神秘伝" in Japanese, meaning "Mystery Teachings") we become a master & we know science of scanning. Reiki 3 is learned just like Reiki-2 in 4 hours. The Reiki 3 healer is known as a Reiki master. This is because he can produce very powerful healing.

Here, the master symbol, along with it, he also learns two additional supporting symbols. He also learns how to scan the patient. Then he can find out exactly where the problem lies.

In this level, a seeker learns about the qualities of a master, this helps a person to unfold the master within himself. He also learns about duties and responsibilities of a master.

In addition, he knows what a master must do and what a master must refrain from. This is necessary as now the Reiki healer does not remain just a channel, he becomes a master.

Now he can create any positive things and events out of his own free will. Till the second degree, the healer just gives Reiki as a channel. He has no power to interfere the plan of the divine.

Now he has the power to create events of his choice and he can create any event he wants. But just as this is very great, it is also very risky. One wrong wish of a master or one wrong statement by a master can even create a disaster. So, a master has to learn how to use this ability in the most responsible way!

If a master behaves in an irresponsible manner, he may cause problems to himself as well as for others. So, a master must be careful in wishing and saying things.

The two additional supporting symbols that he learns here; help the healing happen faster and with greater effect.

One of them is the **SWASTIK OM TRISHOOL** that is quite popular by now. I had received this in the year 1993 from the masters. This has been my registered foundation logo since then. My Reiki students use it since the same time. This is used in the beginning of the healing session.

The other symbol is **EH HE YEH** meaning *I am That*. This symbol is used to keep the patient protected after healing session is over. This symbol is used at the end of the healing session.

With these additional symbols, techniques and knowledge; the Reiki healer gets a new dimension in healing and the master symbol gives him the power to be a creator of the events he chooses. This enhances the healing power of the healer to a very great extent.

DEFINITION OF A MASTER:

Traditionally, a person who uses all the four Reiki symbols including DI KO MYO is called a Reiki master.

Really this is not so. In addition to knowing the master symbol, a master must also have a well developed intuition and connections with the masters from the fifth dimension.

With this, a master can deal with the energies at a much higher level and can produce healing in more effective way.

Masters in the 5th dimensions are all the Gurus that people respect and worship.

There are people who call these masters as angels.

This is the reason why at times you also hear people saying that when you become a Reiki master, you get your guardian angel.

In fact, when we get in touch with the masters, we keep getting guidance from these masters but only a master can read these guidance signals that we get.

Others feel that they must do something, but cannot read the actual signals.

They always guide us, but after becoming a master, you can understand their guidance better.

A Reiki master has a well balanced attitude towards everything. It is this attitude that helps him heal more effectively.

The master develops this attitude as his emotions and attachjments are worked upon during his training as a master.

He learns the importance of the detached attachment.

With this, he has love and affection for everyone, but no expectations of things that he knows he does not really deserve.

Dropping attachments and emotions means; Knowing that whatever you deserve, is certainly going to come to you! It is the law of universe.

Attachment is your connection with things around.

Technically speaking, one cannot survive without attachments at all even for a fraction of a second!

But the attachments are of two kinds. Detached and attached.

Detached attachment is the one that is like I have defined above. When you have detached attachment, you do not expect anything; you just work to deserve it.

You know that once you deserve it, you are anyways going to get it. This means, if you are not getting something that you wish to have, you do not deserve it, and must do something to deserve it.

With this knowledge, master utilizes his time and energy to improve upon him when he wants to have something. This makes him more powerful.

When a person has attached attachment on the other hand, he just wants something, longs for it, expects that someone will come and GIVE it to him, and when this does not happen, gets upset due to pain and frustration.

This is the reason why common men always say that attachment leads to pain. What the spiritual people discourage is this attached attachment.

Emotion is Energy in MOTION.

This means, when our energies start moving on their own due to some excitement, we say we have emotions.

Yet we must know that when we experience emotions, the experience as well as expression is of two types.

In one case, we are in control of emotions, and in the other, emotions are in control of us.

Generally, in the second situation, people say that we are having emotions, but the fact is just the other way; the emotion is having us!

This is a bad situation and master knows how to avoid it.

Master knows that experiencing an emotion is fine. Also, expressing it is fine.

Only losing control over the emotion while doing so is not fine.

Master also knows that if he deserves something, that thing will come to him in any way!

He also knows the value and nuisance value of things like anxiety and judgment.

In spite of being a Reiki channel, some people do not know how to handle some situations and feel powerless.

At such times, a master works quite effectively.

This is because, he knows when to entrust things to the existence.

When harmony cannot be created by human efforts, a master leaves this job to the nature.

He knows that the nature has the power to create harmony everywhere.

May be this is the reason why when we need a break, we prefer to go in the midst of the nature for relaxation!

The master also knows that in our mind, this harmony is lost due to our attachments and emotions.

He knows how to drop the attachments & emotions and restore the harmony within.

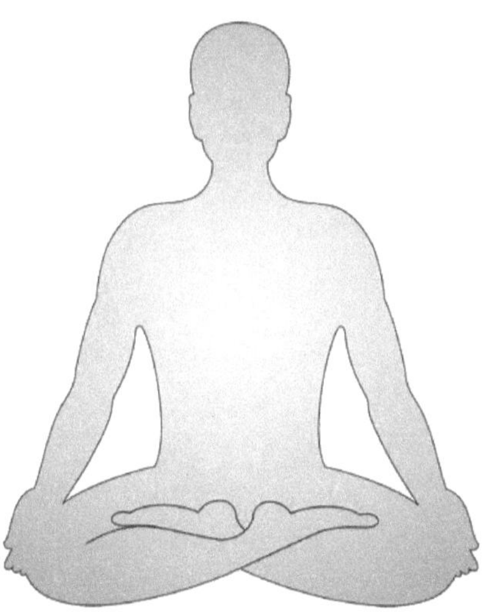

SYMBOLS:

Let us see the symbols that a master must learn:

THE MASTER SYMBOL: DAI KOME YO:

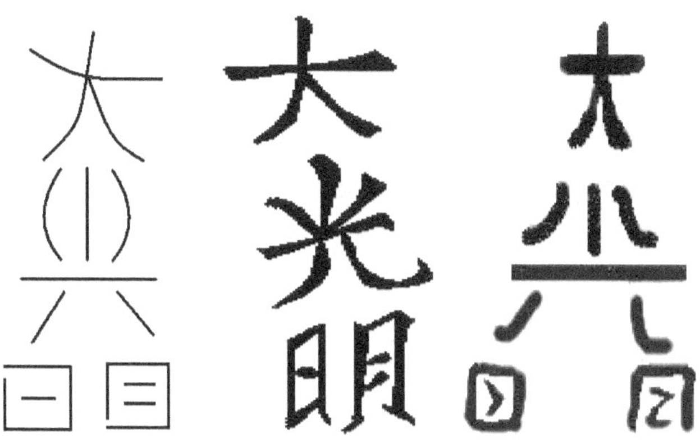

This is the symbol that a master learns in the third degree of Reiki. It gives him the power to create events of his choice by taking the responsibility of results of those events.

This is also called as DI KO MYO by many Reiki Teachers. In fact, DI KO MYO is a very popular name to this symbol here in India.

The master symbol has a number of variations. At least 15 of them are commonly known and taught by different Reiki teachers, as masters write it in many different ways.

After about 20 years of work over finding the Sanskrit mantra for this, I finally got the Sanskrit Mantra for the Master symbol and realised that it is the most used statement in Indian Spiritual world. The Mantra is **"AHAM BRAHMAASMI"** (meaning: I am the supreme creator)

All these variations are equally powerful, so one can use any of the above variation that one finds easy. No variation is right or wrong, no variation is good or bad or correct or incorrect. The variation that I found most workable is given here with detailed explanation:

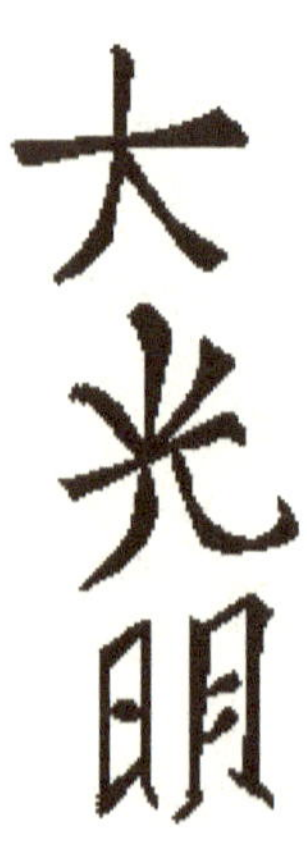

DAI = big man, large or great in Japanese. The lines formation also suggests the connection with the five subtle elements responsible in the production of things.

KOME = growing (rice = event) in the presence of ray of light or brightness that shines, according to one explanation while it means energy protection as per the other.

YO = grounding & creating due to the oneness with the universe. The other meaning of myo is, clear open bright radiance.

Other variations of Dai Kome Yo are as follows:

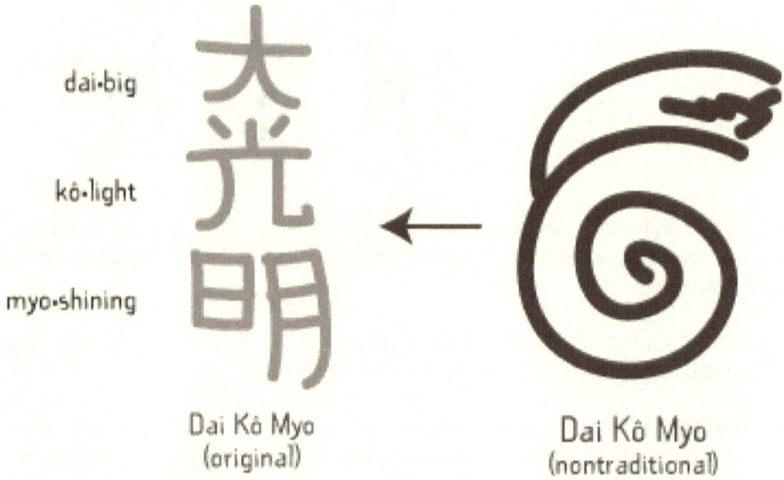

dai·big

kô·light

myo·shining

Dai Kô Myo
(original)

Dai Kô Myo
(nontraditional)

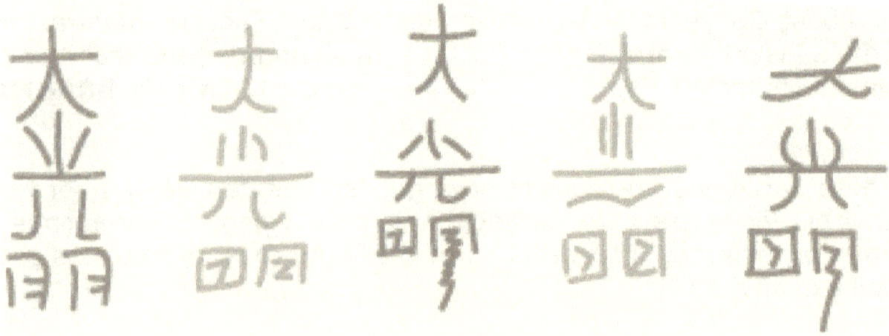

Variants of the original symbol

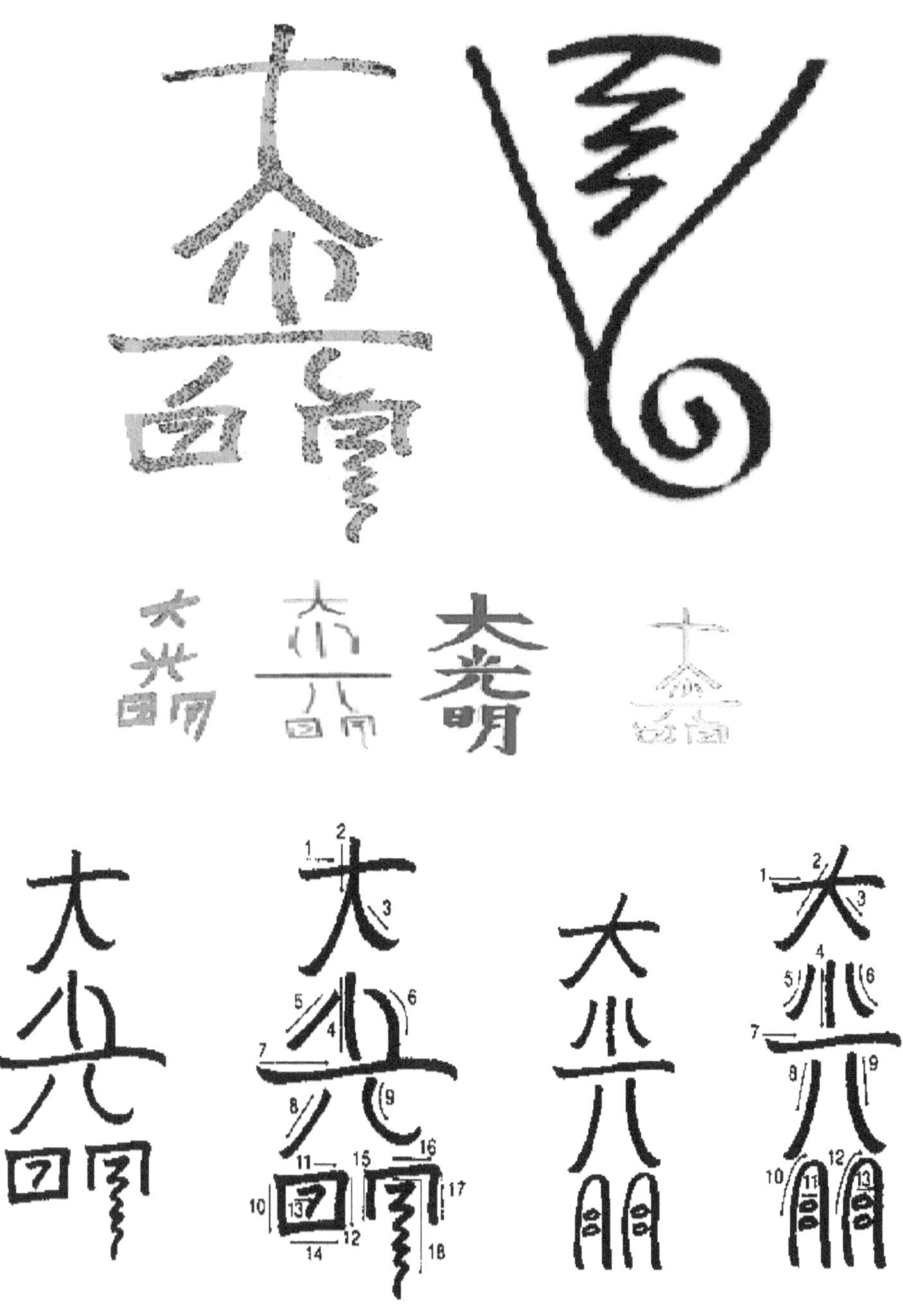

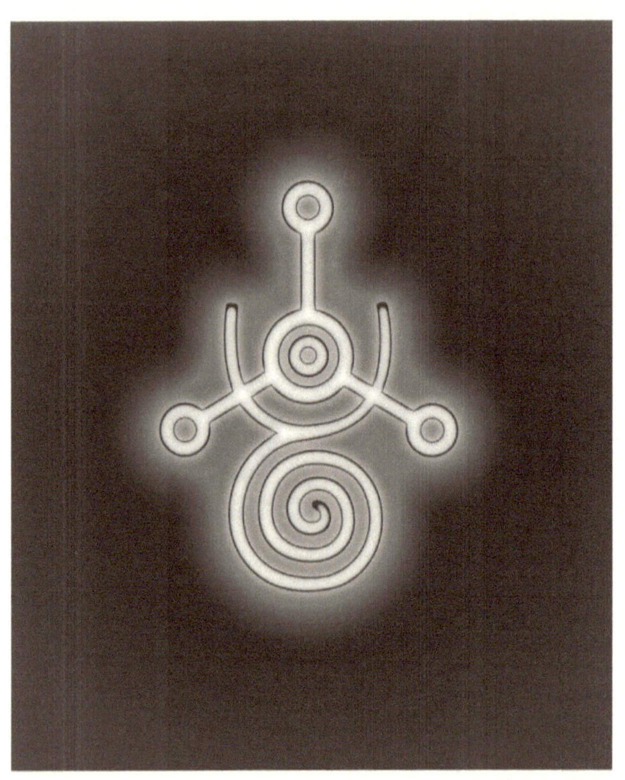
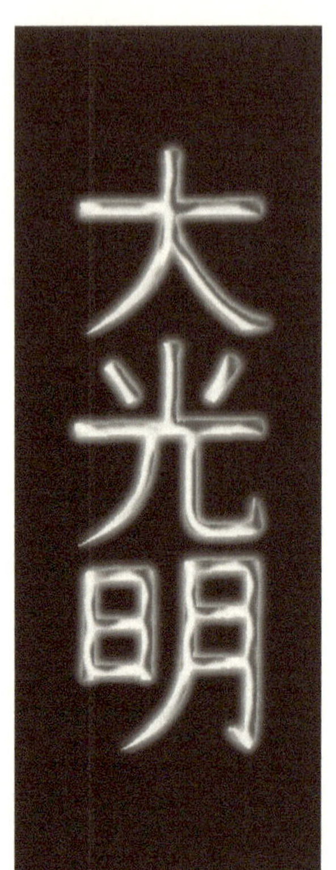
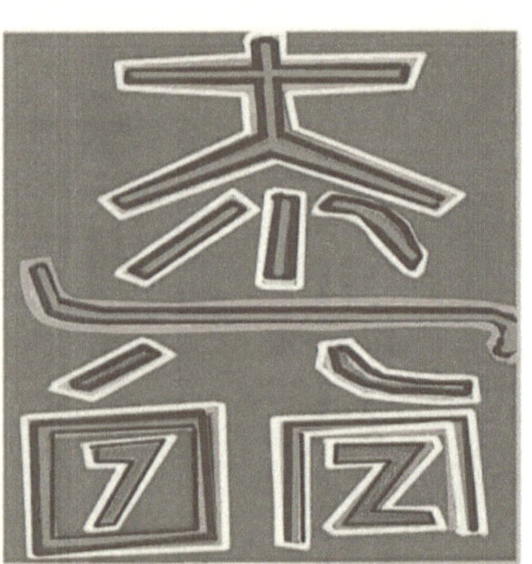
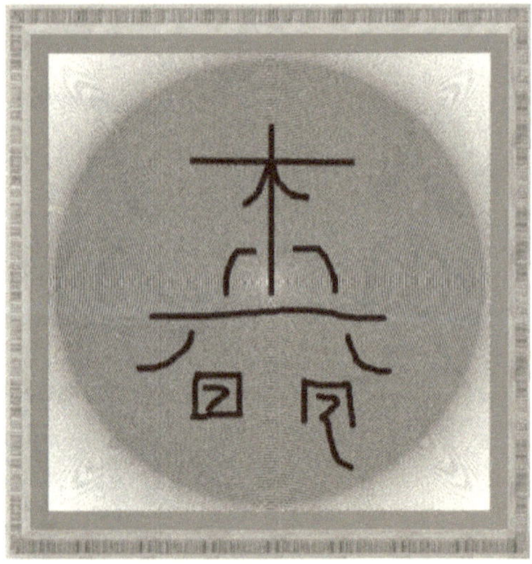

OTHER SUPPORTING SYMBOLS

Along with these traditional symbols, there are two symbols that I have found to be effective. These are, **SWASTIK OM TRISHOOL & EH HE YEH.** They can be used in the beginning and at the end of the healing session as given below.

The **SWASTIK OM TRISHOOL** was received by me in 1993. This is a unique combination of the three traditional symbols. The **Swastik** indicates the **beginning**. It invokes the creator energies. The **OM** indicates the **protection**. It invokes the protecting & sustaining energies. The **trishool** indicates **destruction**. It invokes the destroying energies for the destruction of negative. With these energies at work, healing happens much faster. The Sanskrit Mantra for it is **HAMSAH.**

I recommend the use of this symbol before starting the healing session. As you use this symbol, you invoke the blessings of the CREATOR, PROTECTOR and DESTROYER energies, i.e. the **G**enerator, **O**rganizer, **D**estroyer i.e. the **GOD** energy.

This symbol is recommended to be used before starting the healing session. As you use this symbol, you invoke the blessings of the creator, protector and destroyer energies, i.e. the **G**enerator, **O**rganizer, **D**estroyer i.e. the **GOD** energy.

Also drawing this symbol in the house on the main door in red ink is good to bring good luck and keep bad energies away.

If anyone draws this in red colour on all doors, windows and walls of the house or office, or any premises, that place is protected from all bad energies.

Wearing a locket or charm of this symbol can protect a person from all evils.

All this happens as the energy vibrations that come out of this symbol create a protecting layer around a person or place where the symbol is placed.

Anyone belonging to any religion or nationality can try this and benefit by this.

This being a **siddha symbol**, it does not need any attunement, yet, if one receives it from a master qualified to give it, one gets greater benefit.

Since this information is coming to you all directly from the one who received the symbol, if you read this and use this symbol, you will certainly get 100% benefit of the symbol!

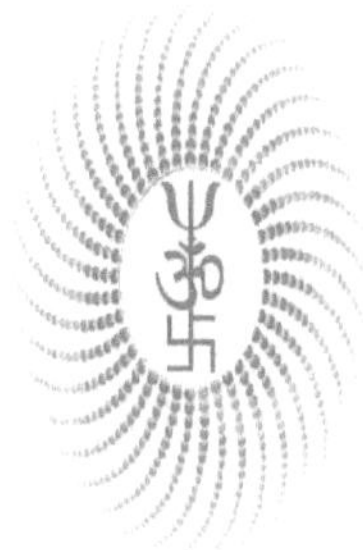

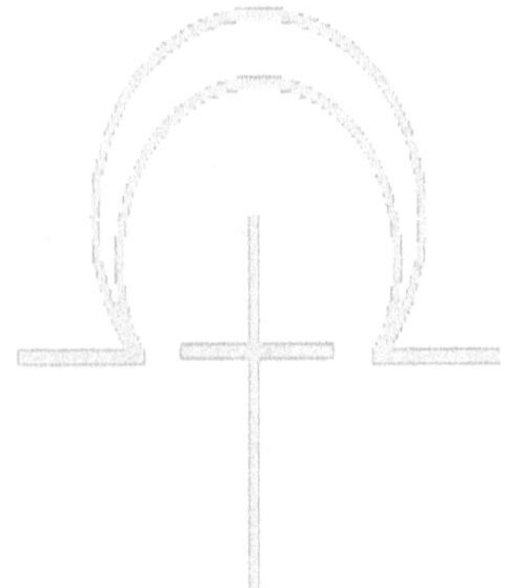

The other symbol that I recommend here is, **EH HE YEH**.

The meaning of this symbol as I got is, 'I AM THAT (universal energy)'.

In Sanskrit, it is called **SOHAM**.

When you draw this symbol while concluding the Reiki treatment, you keep the patient connected with the universal energies even after the treatment so that whenever patient needs Reiki later before next healing session, he keeps getting it from universe.

Also, protective shield of this symbol prevents loss of energies received by patient. This symbol is drawn in fluorescent green colour. This is the colour of heart chakra. Also, it signifies green fire that burns negative energies.

When you draw this symbol after healing session, the clairvoyant people can see that it settles around the person, thing or event healed.

The white vertical line covers the patient, thing or event healed. The green horizontal line turns into a ring that protects this person, thing or event covered by the white vertical line.

Further, the hat like structure, made up of fluorescent green gives a stronger and lasting protection shield to this person, thing or event healed.

If one wants, one may also visualise such a three dimensional EH HE YEH. But since this imagination is a bit complicated, I suggest the students to just draw it as it is at the end of every healing session.

At times, this symbol is seen to be used by the Buddhist people with a very powerful prayer; NAM MYOHO RENGE KYO. This is a very popular prayer of nichiren-shoshu-Buddhism.

In Bible and Jewish literature too we find references of the term used as Eh He Yeh meaning I am that.

These additional supporting symbols prove to be very useful in healing with traditional symbols.

Generally, I advise the healers to *begin* the healing session with SWASTIK OM TRISHOOL & *conclude* it with EH HE YEH.

This helps the healer to get the healing started faster as well as get the patient protected after healing is over.

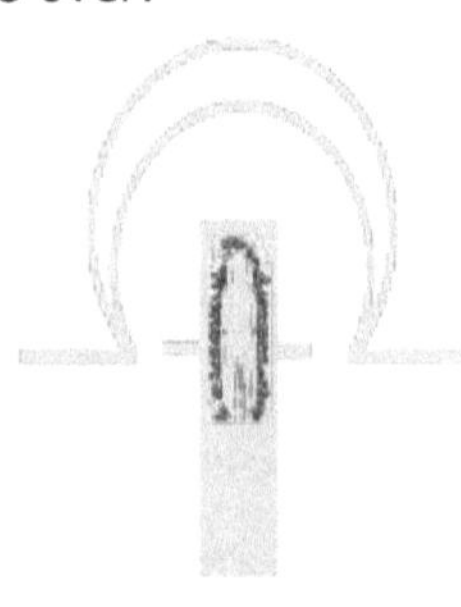

MAIN PROCEDURE FOR THE USE OF SYMBOLS:

@ **Visualize, see** or **imagine** the *affected person, animal, area of the body, the object or the machine, the event you wish to create, thought you want to change, past thought, spirit you want to heal*. Or **write** the **intention** on a paper. Put it in a **box**.

@ Make your vision as clear as possible. If you are visualizing or imagining, add as many details as you can to the image you visualize, so that the image will be almost complete as you want it to be. (In common language, this is called *covering* the person, body part, animal, image or object *with white light*)

@ Mentally draw Reiki symbols over the visualized image in the following order:

@ Draw ⟊ Mentally over the imagined image in red or orange

@ Draw 大光明 Say Dai kome yo 3 times.

@ Draw 本字人 Say hon sha zai sho nen 3 times / say HONG SAHA JOOM SAHA NAMAH 3 times

@ Draw Say se hei ki 3 times / say HASKLEEM NAMAH 3 times

@ Draw Say chokkou rei 3 times / say CHAKRE 3 times

@ **Mentally give Reiki till you feel the vibrations or heat.**

◎ Mentally draw symbols again over image with desired change.

◎ Draw 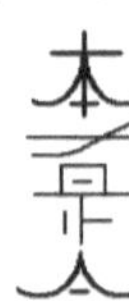 Say Dai kome yo 3 times.

◎ Draw 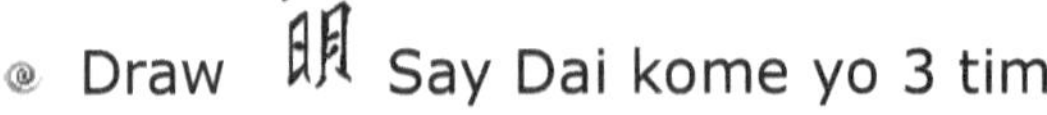 Say hon sha zai sho nen 3 times / say HONG SAHA JOOM SAHA NAMAH 3 times

◎ Draw Say se hei ki 3 times / say HASKLEEM NAMAH 3 times

◎ Draw Say chokkou rei 3 times / say CHAKRE 3 times

◎ Draw 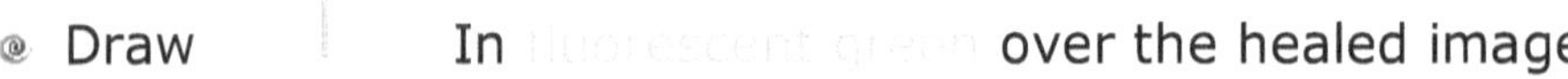 In fluorescent green over the healed image

◎ **Request Reiki to keep working till the event or thing needs energy to materialize the desired change and stop.**

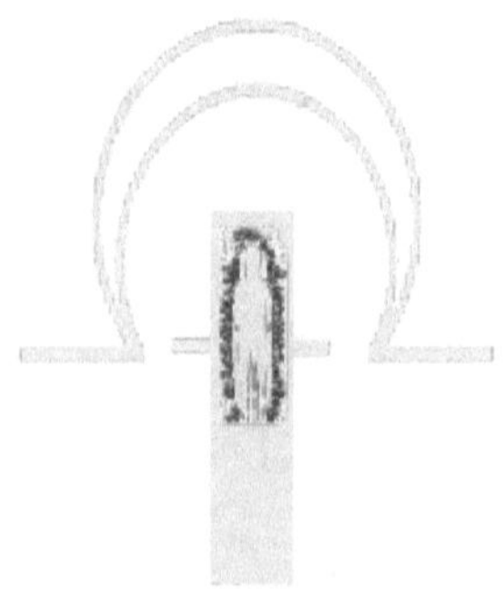

111

DO LIKE THIS:

Imagine and draw;

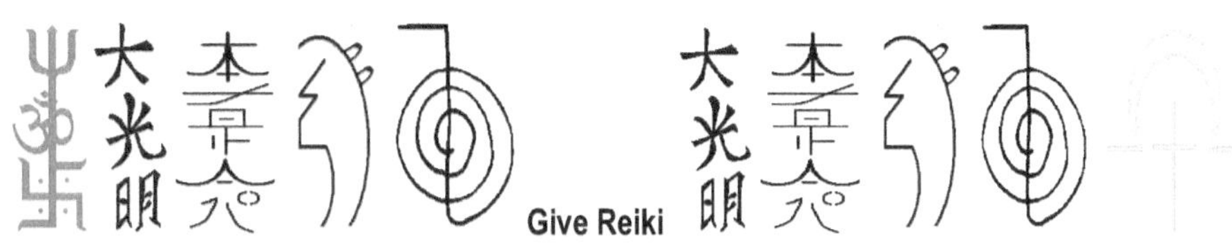

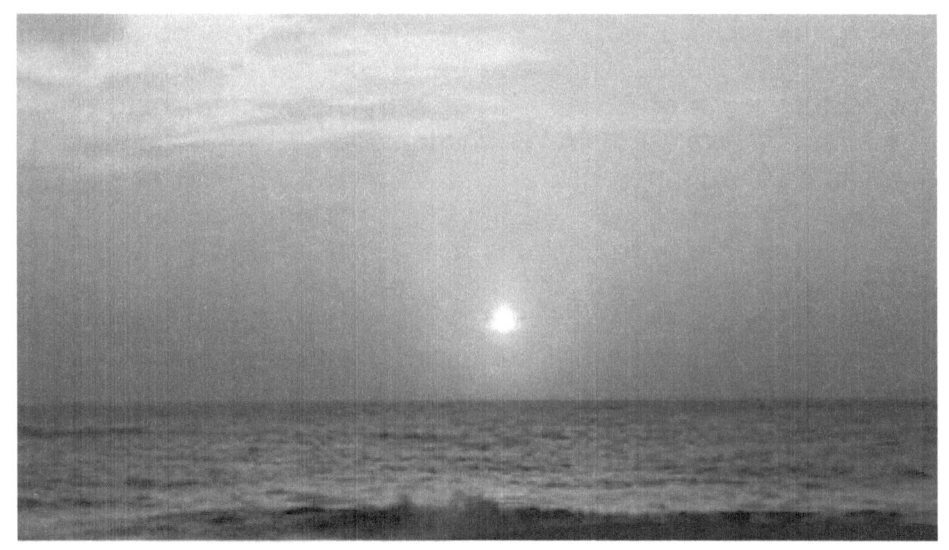

MIND BODY RELATION:

We all know that a healthy mind stays in a healthy body and vice versa. If mind loses health, the body becomes unhealthy in some time. Similarly, if body is unhealthy, mind becomes irritable.

It is medically proved that 99% of the ailments originate in the mind. So, when we know the psychology of ailments, we can remove the root cause of it from the mind, both with Reiki and counselling.

A good Reiki healer must remember that he has to remove the root cause of problem. If a person is sick, it is because, he has invited the sickness subconsciously for some payoff. We must make a patient aware of this without offending him and make his mind clear that he need not invite ailment for he is not going to get any benefit by that.

This means, we must talk to him and also provide him some counselling that can help him locate, accept and then release the thoughts and emotions that have made him sick. When we do this successfully, Reiki works faster and the ailment once healed, does not recur. We know that even the most dreaded ailment like cancer recurs a few years, even after chemo therapy, when root cause from mind of patient is not removed. Same thing happens in many ailments, and so, removing roots of the ailment from the mind is absolutely necessary.

For doing this, we find out the problem a patient is having and conclude the type of thought or emotion that is bugging him. Generally, any part of the body gets affected after about 6 months from the time of getting a shock. So, when a patient approaches, on seeing the symptoms, a healer may refer to the table of emotions and body parts and ask the patient relevant questions.

From the answers, the healer may get to know how much he is accurate. Then he can also start combining various Reiki methods to heal the patient quickly and effectively.

EMOTION & BODY CONNECTION:

BODY PART	EMOTION	BODY PART	EMOTION
FOREHEAD	IMAGINATION & INTELLECTUAL ISSUES	FOREARM	SELF ESTEEM & SUCCESS
EYES	PERCEPTION OF THE WORLD	UPPER ARM	STRENGTH & COURAGE
BROWS	INTUITION & EMOTIONAL EXPRESSION	HANDS	GIVING, GETTING, REACHING GOALS & WORKABILITY
NOSE	SELFRECOGNITION & SELF-IMAGE	CHEST	RELATIONSHIP, LOVE, WARMTH
EARS	LISTENING & HEARING	HEART	LOVE & AFFECTION
JAWS	VERBAL EXPRESSION	DIAPHRAGM	POWER OF WISDOM
MOUTH	SURVIVAL, SECURITY & ACCEPTANCE OF NEW IDEAS	ABDOMEN	STORAGE OF EMOTIONS
FACE	ATTITUDE TO LIFE	GENITALS	SURVIVAL
THROAT	EXPRESSION	THIGHS	STRENGTH & SELF-TRUST
NECK	MIXTURE OF THOUGHTS, EMOTIONS & EXPRESSION	KNEES	FEAR OF DEATH & CHANGE
SHOULDERS	RESPONSIBILITY	LOWER LEGS	GOAL-DIRECTED ACTIONS
UPPER BACK	ANGER	ANKLES	BALANCE IN BEHAVIOUR
LOWER BACK	TENSION OF EMOTION	FEET	COMPETITION, ABILITY & DESIRE TO REACH GOAL

Remember the above table thoroughly in order to be able to analyze the emotions behind every problem.

SCANNING

Scanning is finding out what is the problem with the system; let it be a physical body, or event or anything like machine.

As we scan something, we are trying to find out what is wrong with that thing or person or object. This is possible when we mentally see any object and try to know the area of its problem.

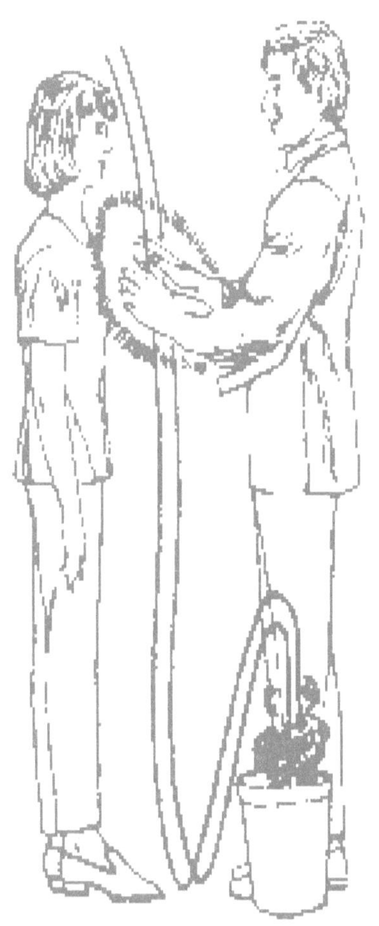
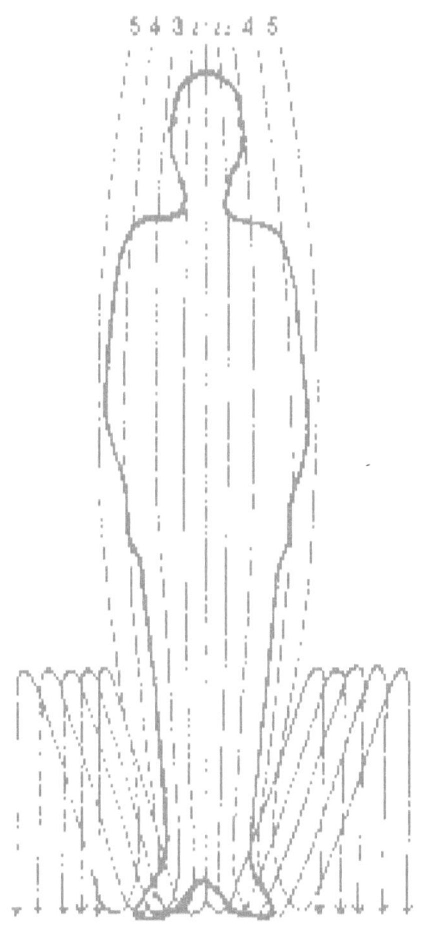

To do this we need to keep the eyes closed. Then we need to bring the thing that we want to scan in front of our eyes. As we do this, the problem is seen in a clear way.

First concentrate your mind. Then think of the thing that you want to heal. Now bring the image of that object in front of your eyes. In the beginning you may need to close your eyes and imagine.

When you scan a person, begin with the head and go down looking for problem. The Area with problem would be different from the rest of the body. Make a note of it. Like this see the entire body of the patient from front and back.

After you finished ask the patient about his problems and see whether you were right. Afterwards you can heal the patient. You need to do this to a number of patients till the time you are perfect.

When you are checking an object for its mechanical fault, it is advisable that the mechanism is studied before you scan. When you do this, you won't be making errors in your judgment. You can then mentally study the entire machine and you'll know the area of problem quite easily which you may check with the expert again.

When you are checking an event, try to study all possible situations that create that event, only then start analyzing the event. This would give you a greater insight into the event that you are working on. With this insight, you will be in a better position to find out the exact cause of the problem. You can practice scanning the persons, objects as well as events in this way.

When you do this, you need to feel energies with hands and must have your hands ready to feel these energies. By practicing Reiki regularly, one certainly gets this sensitivity, yet, there are some simple steps to make your hands sensitive to touch the aura and scan effectively. These are:

1. Press the centre of your palms by thumb.
2. Press the fingers of both hands gently.
3. Rotate the hands clockwise & counter clockwise.
4. Slowly increase distance between hands & feel pull
5. Now your hands are ready to touch aura & scan.

See the figures below to know how this is to be done:

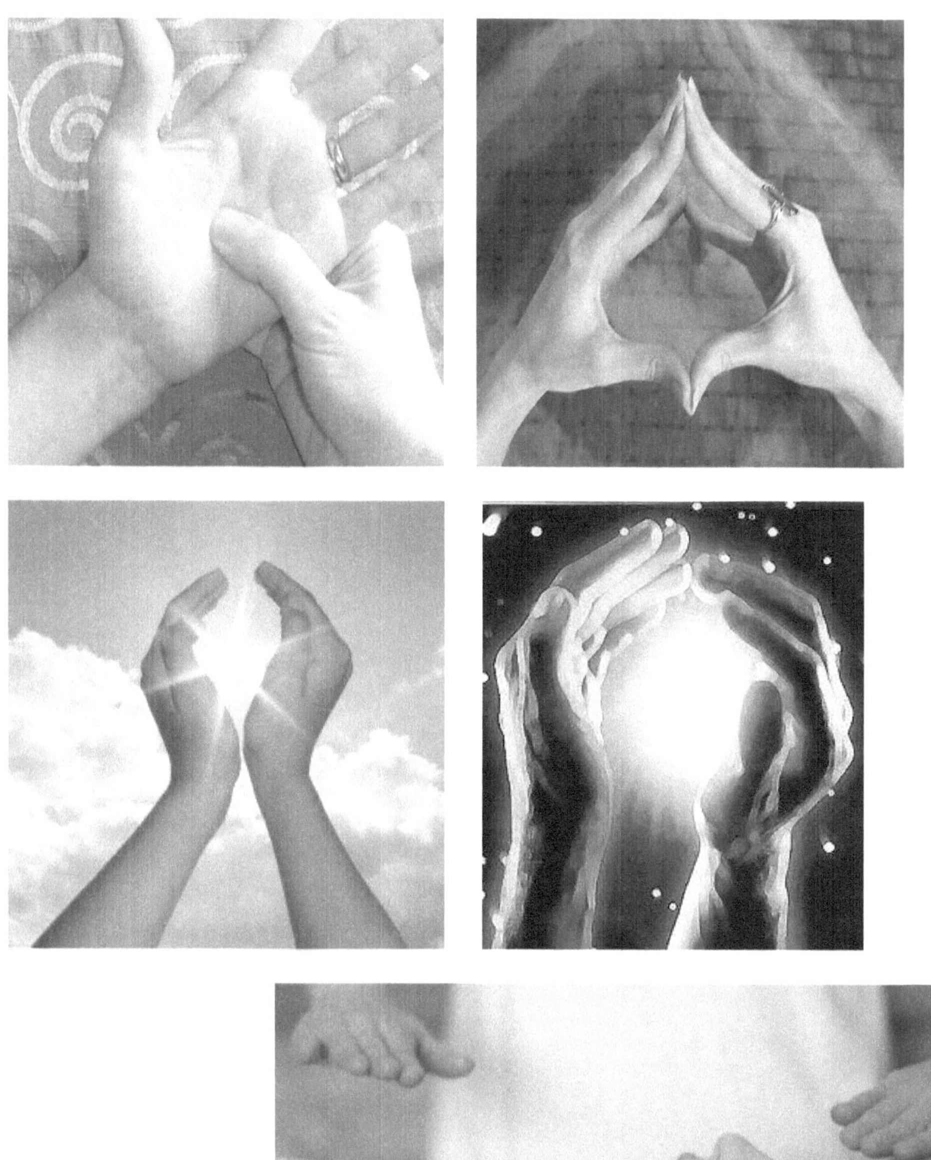

CHAKRAS IN AURA:

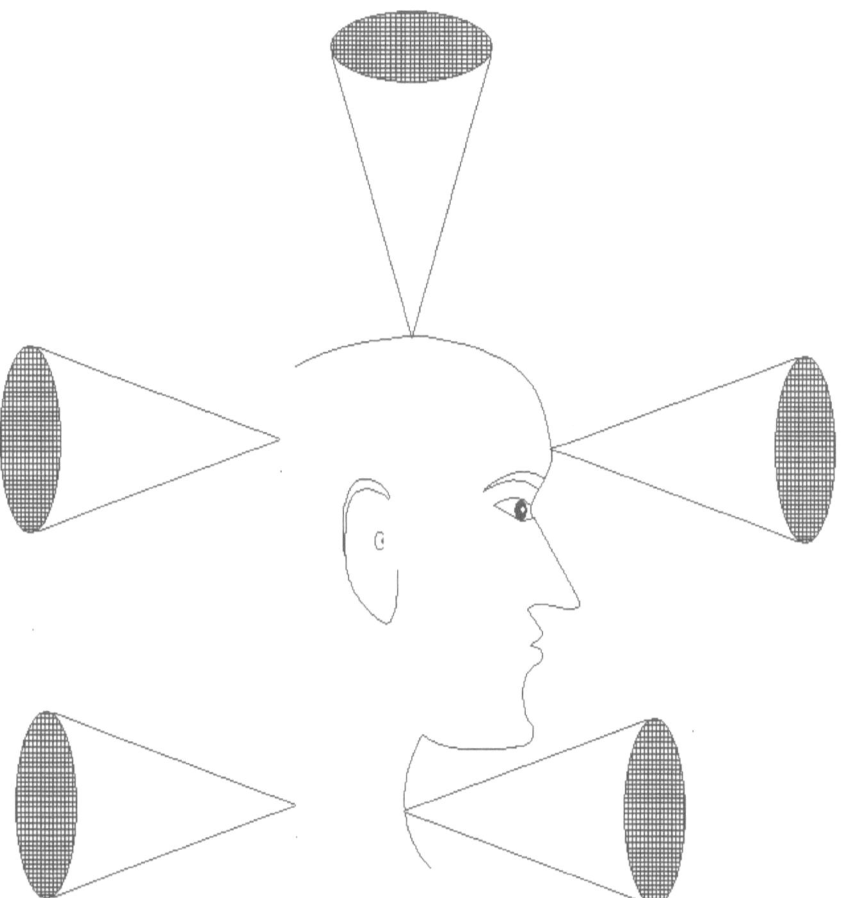

Chakras look somewhat like the above image in our aura. Clairvoyant persons and those who have learned Aura healing can see them with normal eyes. Others can just feel them with hands after Reiki 3 training. But they are there in every person's aura.

This is the reason why when we move our hands a few inches away from the body of a person, we can feel the aura and chakras at around the distance of about 4 to 5 inches.

When we are checking the distance of aura, we feel the touch at this distance. Also the person whom you are scanning feels the touch.

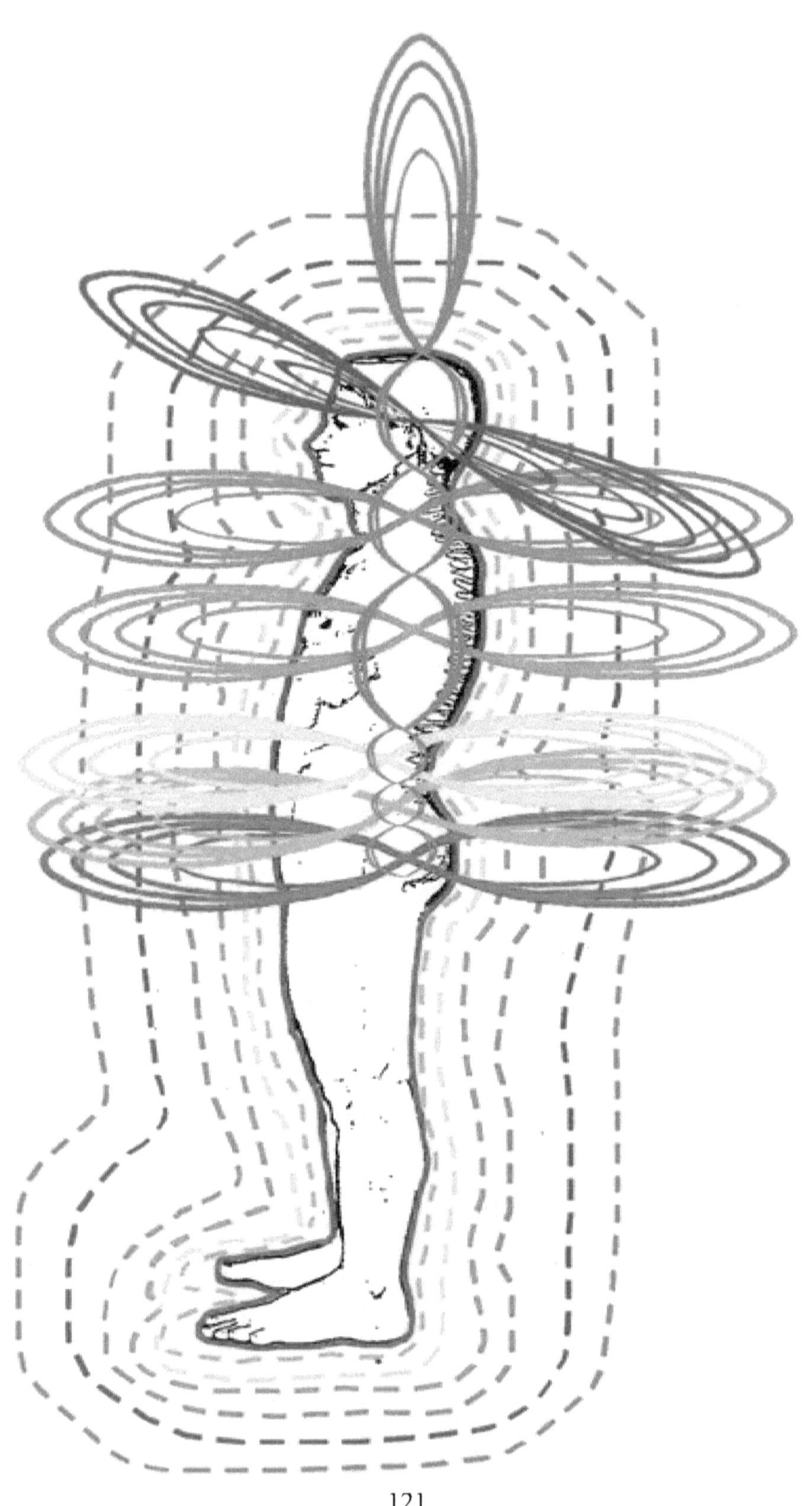

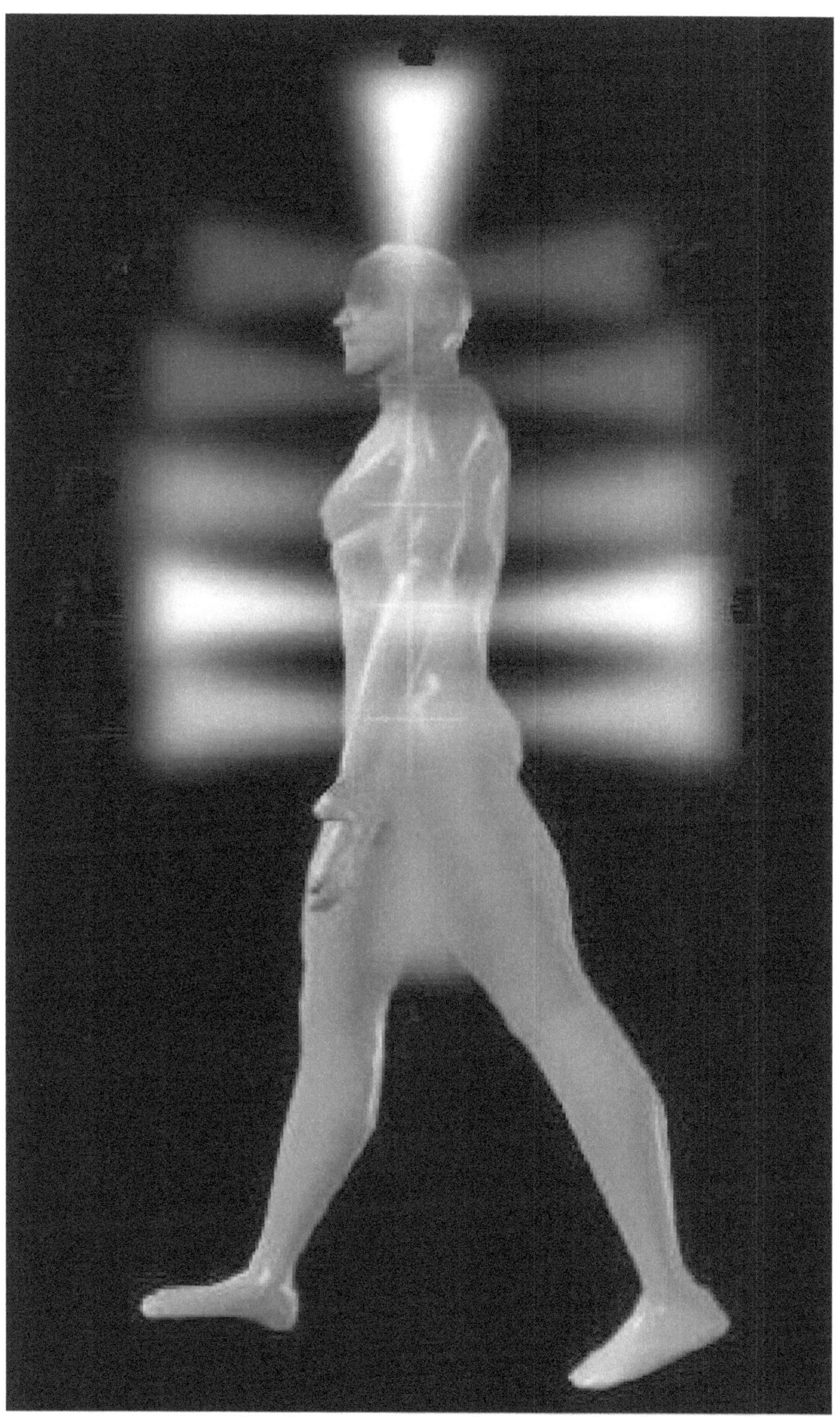

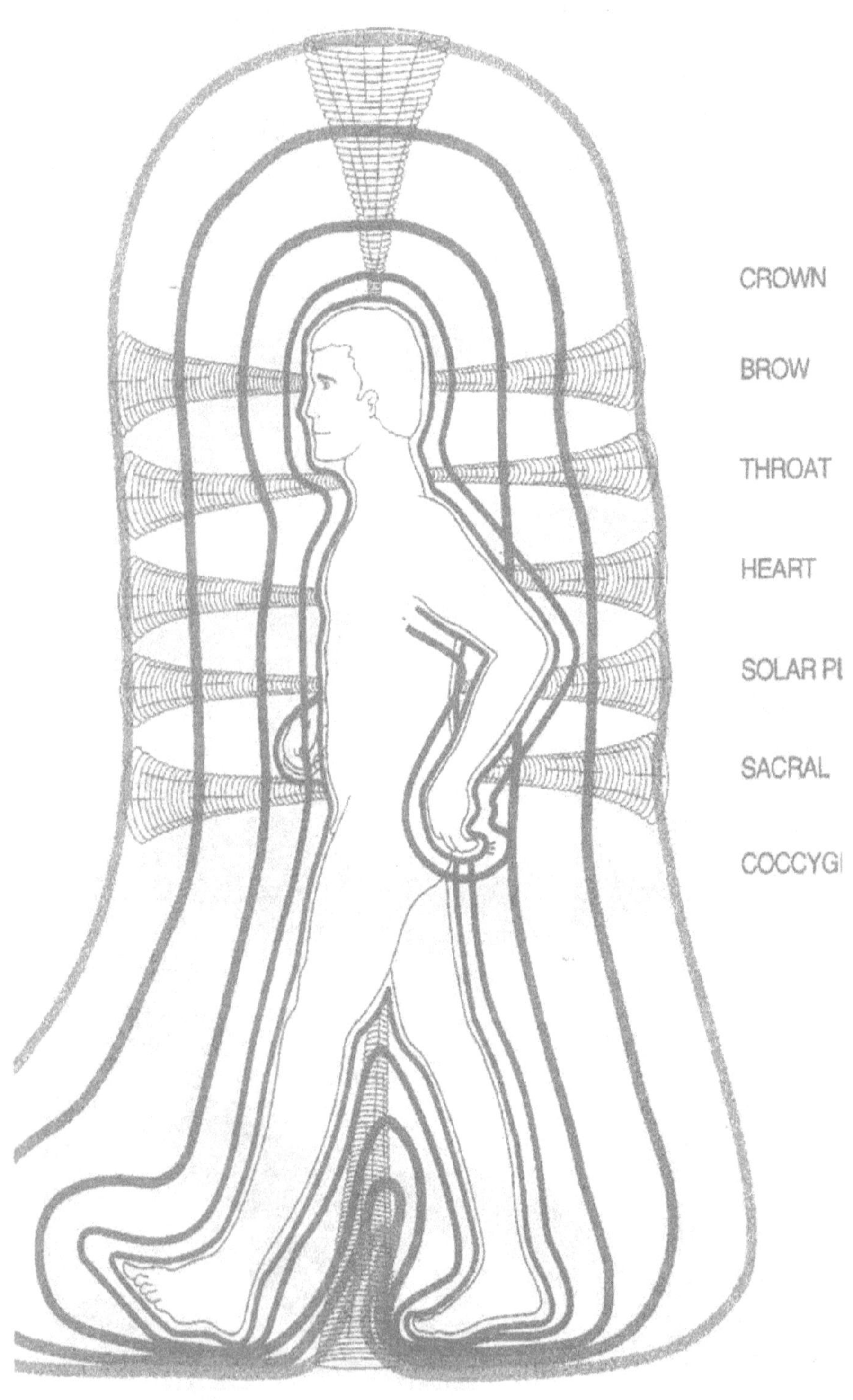

CROWN
BROW
THROAT
HEART
SOLAR PL
SACRAL
COCCYG

Chakras look like this when healthy:

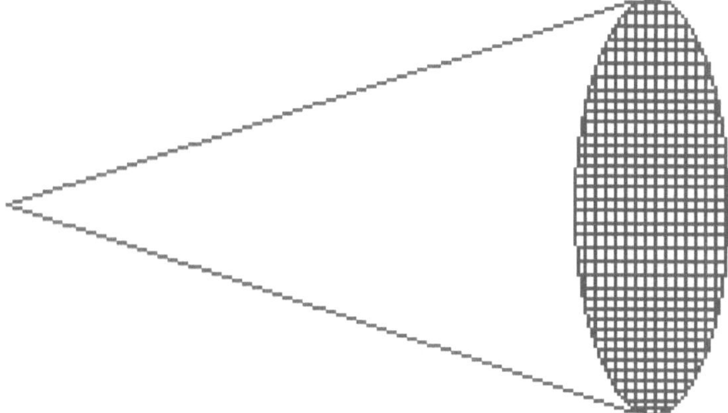

But when their covering shield gets weaker, they look like this:

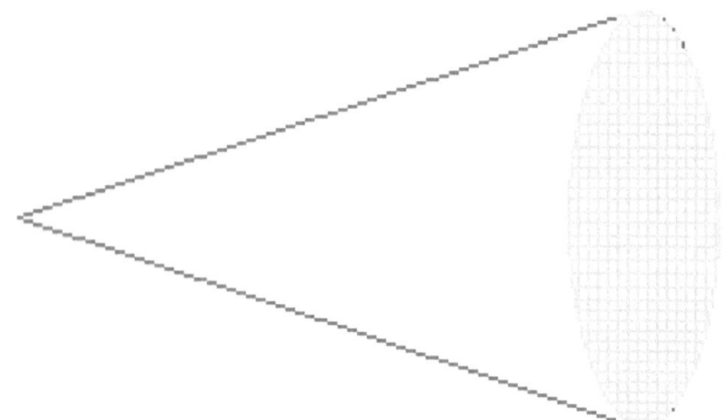

When this net breaks, they look like this:

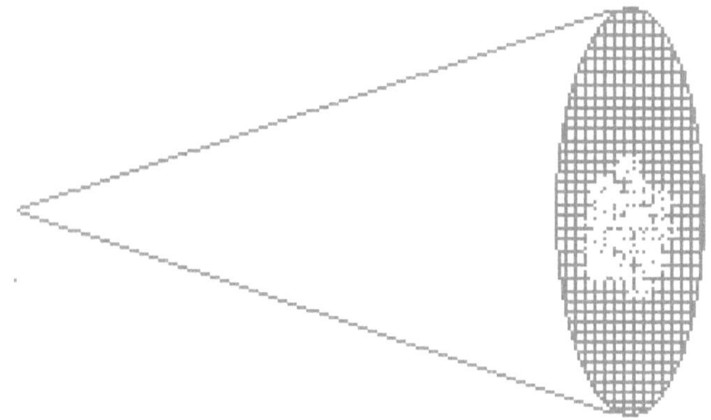

When they have dirt in them, they look like this:

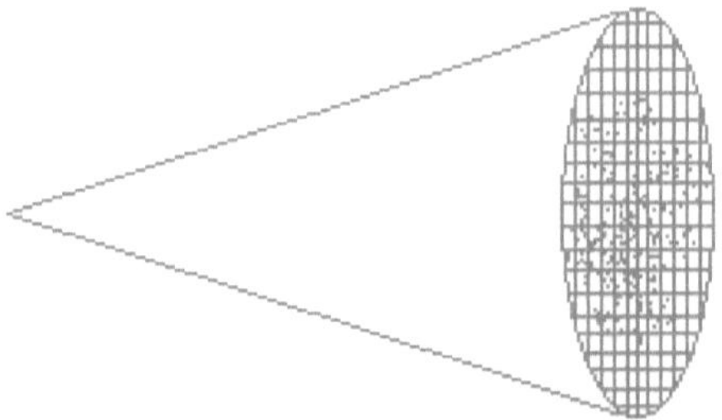

When the dirt is more, they look like this:

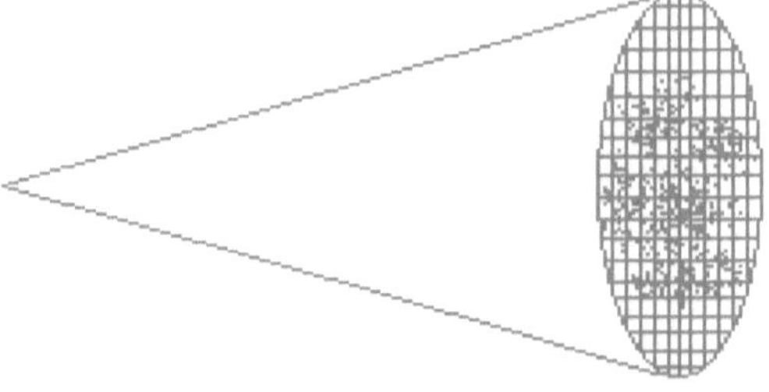

When there are negative elementals attached into them, they look like this:

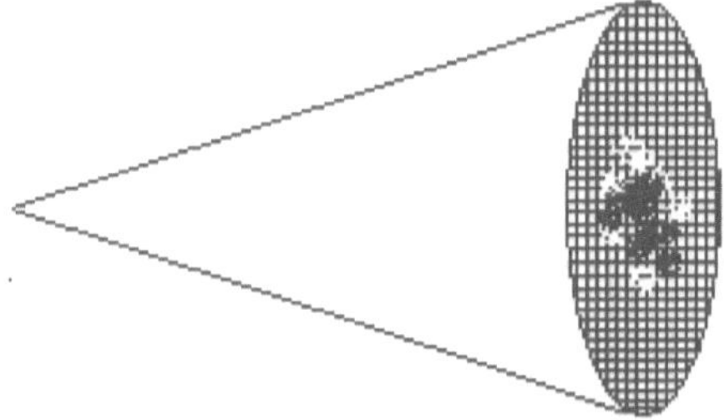

If there is a psychic attack, the chakra looks somewhat like this:

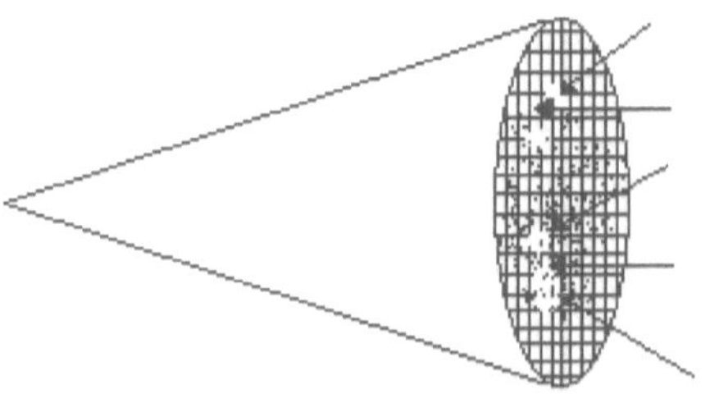

SICK CHAKRAS

The sick chakras look somewhat like this:

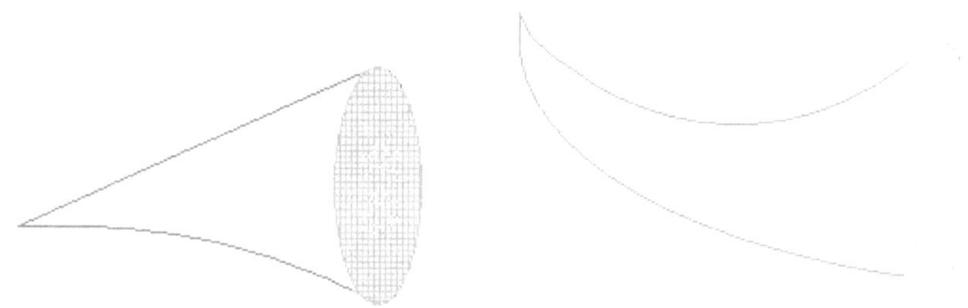

When a person is in a double mind, chakras look something like this:

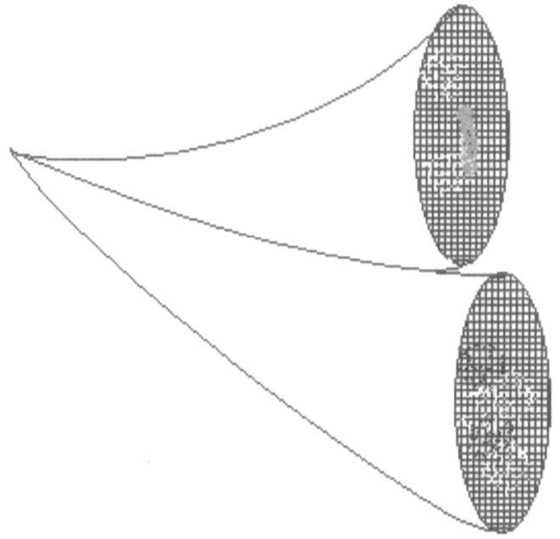

If there is depression along with double mind, chakra looks something like this:

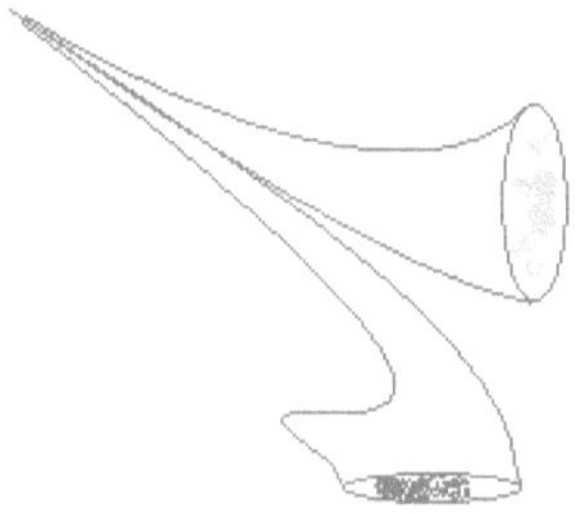

Chakras on hands

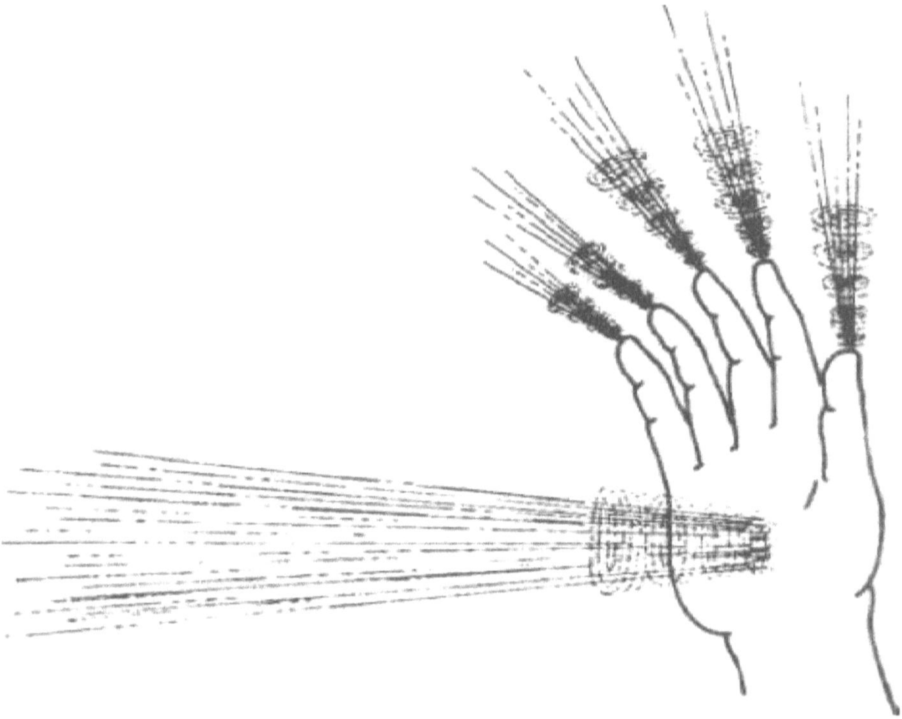

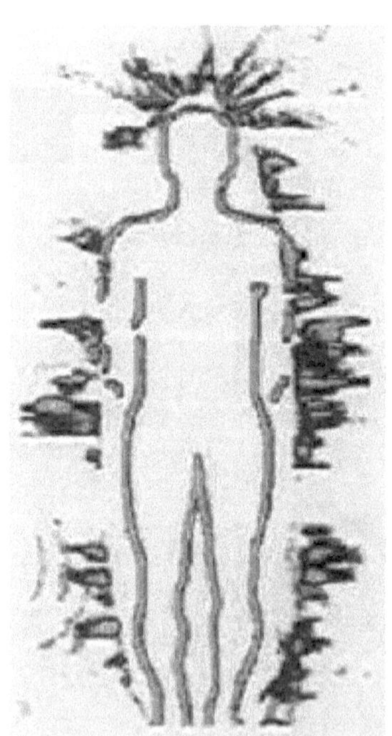

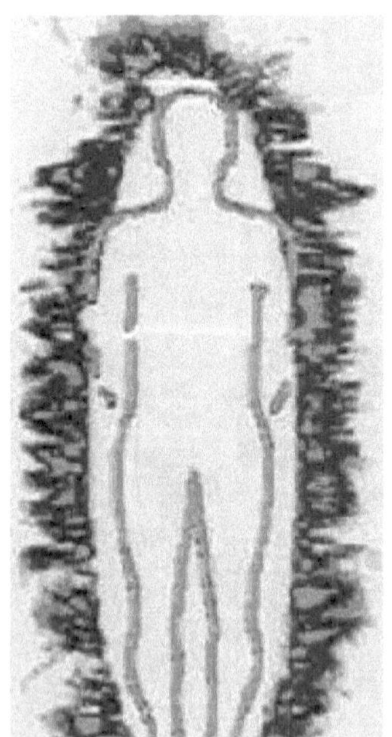

Sick aura   **Healthy aura**

To scan the chakras, we must look for the position of chakras in the positions seen in the image above.

Just like the face, as shown in the image, we find other chakras in related areas on the body.

Check the aura like this and clean the chakras or area that you find having more vibrations.

You can do this by using the aura loosening method that you learned in Reiki 2.

Then check it once again and also ask the feelings of the person whom you are scanning.

If the person reports lighter feeling and absence of pain that he had earlier, know that cleaning is done.

Now, give Reiki to that area, then give Reiki to the whole person by short form method of healing and then give protection and stop.

In this manner you can scan and heal all the chakras.

Once all the chakras are cleaned and healed, give Reiki to the patient for 5 minutes using the short form of Reiki as you do in Reiki 2, while using all the symbols that we use for Reiki 3.

This will heal the patient totally.

Then draw golden Se hei ki on all the 6 sides of the patient as shown in aura loosening of Reiki 2.

After this, draw orange Swastika Om Trishool on all the 6 sides of the patient.

After this is done, visualise a three dimensional Eh He Yeh and place the patient inside it for continued protection.

The three dimensional Eh He Yeh looks some what like this:

The straight vertical line is a beam of white light inside which you visualise the patient.

The horizontal line is a green circle that comes at the heart level of the patient, protecting his heart.

The Hat like structure is like a Green Hat that covers the chakras from above and protects the patient.

Once this is done, you can know that for 24 hours, the patient stays protected and you need to scan him again only after 24 hours when the energies start dissolving.

This scanning and healing makes healing process faster and more effective.

Also, one can know where actually the problem is and then heal it accurately

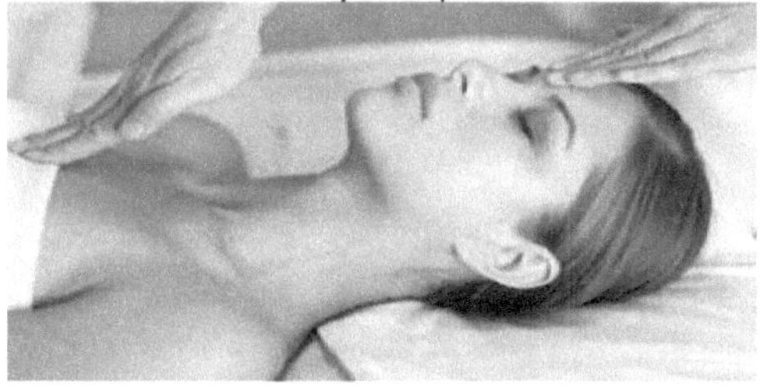

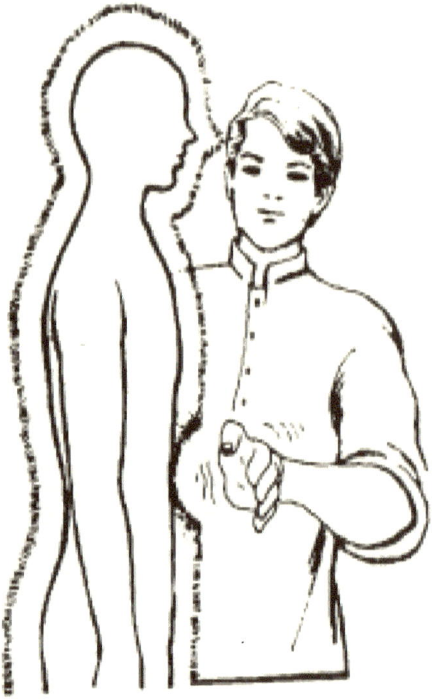

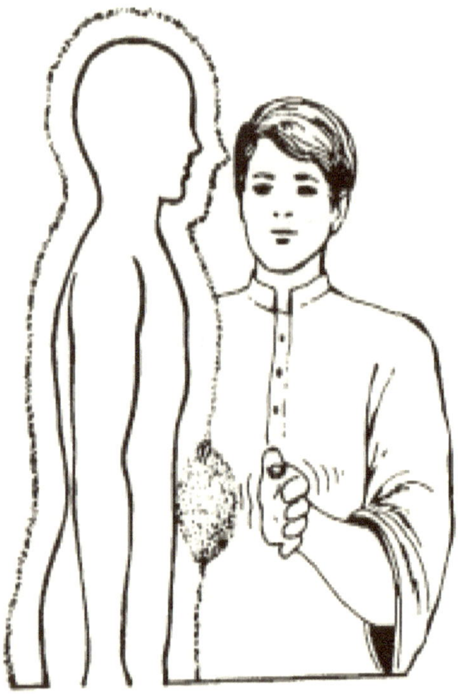

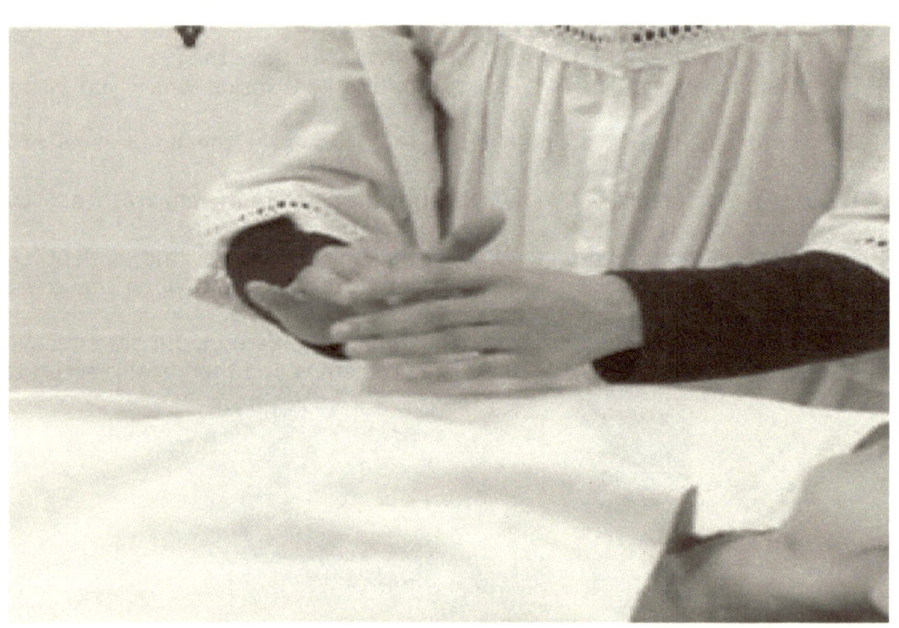

Scanning method helps us to know problem area in anything that we want to heal. We learn to heal scanning here in Reiki 3.

But just this much does not let us heal as a master.

There are many other things that we must do as a master when we heal.

Let us see which these things are:

1: Checking patient's resistance level: Healing is obstructed most of the times due to the resistance a patient has towards getting well.

Many times a person says that he wants to come out of a situation, but actually, he is happy within with the pay-off that he is getting out of that problem.

So he does not want to let go of the pay-off and yet, to satisfy his ego, or to fulfill the social demands, he says that he wants to get rid of the problem.

At such times, it is the duty of the master to check if it is worth releasing the resistance or it is better to let the person be with the problem.

2: Checking our gut feeling: This is when a master has to check his gut feeling.

When a master finds anything or person that needs healing, he must keep his hands on his naval and check the energy he feel there.

This helps a master know his inner attitude towards the person or event or thing to be healed as well as the signals masters are giving about healing that thing.

3: Releasing blocks in patient: if the master feels that he must release the blocks within the patient about healing, the master must begin with that first.

It is only after this is done, a master must start with actual scanning and healing of problem narrated by patient.

4: Checking of the possibility of reoccurrence of problem: Even when we have healed the problem as a master, we find that after a while, the problem appears again.

This happens not just in case of healing with Reiki and other spiritual sciences, but also happens in case of treatments with universally recognized and accepted methods.

This especially happens in ailments like cancer that relapses a few years after chemotherapy or surgery.

So, when a Reiki master heals from master level, he must check the possibility of relapse before finally declaring that the patient is healed.

If he finds the possibility of relapse, he must continue the healing for some more time so that the possibility of relapse is pushed away.

Yet, in some cases, a master must also advice the patient to learn Reiki himself at least till second level and keep healing himself at least twice a week.

PROTECTING AS A MASTER:

Scanning helps us know the problem area and heal it quickly and effectively, but when healing is done, there is a possibility that these negative energies that are released from the system of a patient during the healing process; may get attracted back into the system of a patient in some time.

This may happen if the patient attracts the negativity himself or if some near and dear person of the patient attracts it due to his worry for the patient or if the negative energy has some inner power to re-enter the aura of the patient and produce the problem again.

Yet in any such case, a patient of Reiki Master can stay protected from this possibility if master keeps him under Reiki protection shield for 24 hours till he gives the next healing session to the patient.

For doing this, a master must do a very simple thing after healing is done and after finding that the energies of the patient are now in perfect place.

Following are the steps for making a protection shield:

1. Visualize a transparent ball of fluorescent green light.
2. Visualize the patient inside that ball.
3. Visualize a cover of indigo colour around this ball.
4. Visualize a cover of violet flame around this indigo shield.
5. Visualize a cover of golden light around the violet flame.
6. Visualize golden light emitting Fluorescent Green flame.
7. Visualise the golden light emitting Violet flame around.
8. Let patient be inside this structure till next healing session.

Once a master protects the patient in this way, a master can ensure that released negatives are not attracted back in the patient. This makes the healing by a master very effective and people healed by a master get better results.

Ideally, a Reiki master must protect his patient this way after every healing session so that the healing given by him has a lasting effect. After a number of daily healing sessions in a difficult case, a master may keep such a shield even for a week or so when the patient has become relatively stable and is out of danger.

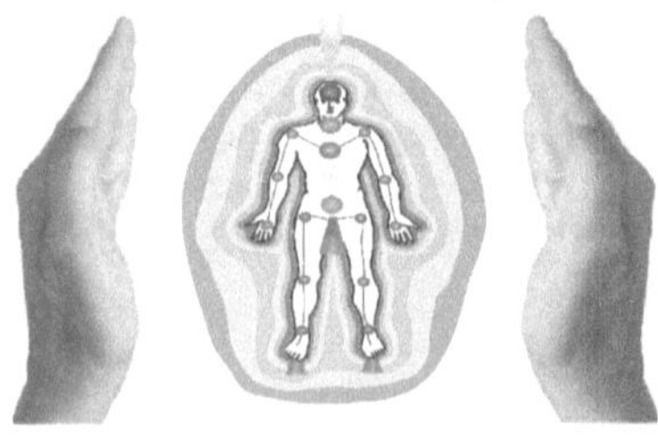

- **MASTER HAS TOTAL CONTROL OVER HIMSELF.**
This means, a master can control bodily demands so effectively, that at times, others do not even realise those demands. For example, of one feels hungry at a place where no food is available, master just gives Reiki to his stomach and his hunger is taken care of, and no one even knows that he was hungry!

- **MASTER SEES NO DIFFERENCE BETWEEN SELF & OTHERS.**
Master is a person without double standards. A double standard is having one rule for oneself & other for others. Master has the same rules for himself & others; there is no difference between himself & others. So whatever is right for himself is right for all, & whatever is wrong for himself is wrong for all in his eyes.

- **MASTER IS ONE WITH THE SURROUNDINGS.**
He can adjust in any situation in the best possible way. A master has no adjustment problems and so blends well everywhere. As a result, a master generally is so transparent that people may find it difficult to differentiate him from any other ordinary person. The only difference between an ordinary person and a master is that a master never complains, he is never unhappy or uncomfortable in any situation whatsoever.

- **MASTER IS IN TOTAL CONTROL OF THOUGHTS EMOTIONS & DESIRES IN HIS MIND.**
A master is fully in control while experiencing as well as expressing emotion as he has this basic knowledge, that losing control over yourself is giving your strings in the hands of others. These others are the ones due to whom the emotion is generated. Once you give your strings in the hands of others, you just become a puppet and then others may take any type of undue advantage of you! A master never lets this happen. He is always in control of himself.

- **MASTER CAN MAKE A POSITIVE DIFFERENCE IN THE LIFE OF OTHERS JUST BY HIS BEING.**
At times, just the presence of a master is enough to heal the person or situation. This is because; the aura of a master is so strong that once anyone enters it, he gets healed.

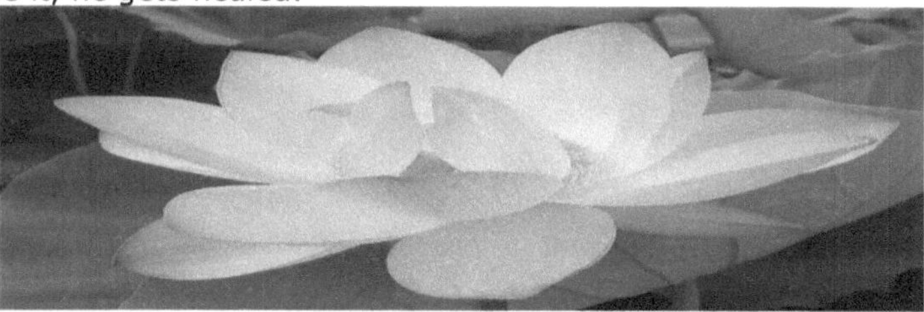

- **A MASTER CAN SCAN A PATIENT AND FIND OUT THE AREA OF PROBLEM. HE CAN DO SO BY MENTALLY SEEING THE AURA OR SCANNING IT WITH HIS HANDS.**
  In the masters' training, one learns to scan a patient or a situation and find out the problem area. Once he learns this, he heals much faster as now he knows what & how much to heal.

- **A MASTER CAN DETECT THE EMOTION INVOLVED IN THE AILMENT FROM OBSERVATION OF SYMPTOMS OF THE PATIENT.**
  A master learns to read, understand and effectively use the chart of emotions and body parts connected with them to know the emotions behind any ailment.

- **A MASTER CAN HEAL THOUGHTS AND EMOTIONS OF A PATIENT.**
  Once a master knows about the emotions involved in the ailment, he can use effective counselling along with Reiki to remove the emotions from the mind of the patient and also he heals the thoughts by using mental method of healing. He knows that 99.99 ailments have a psycho-somatic origin. So along with the body, mind also has to be healed for a permanent recovery.

- **A MASTER CAN CREATE DESIRE IN PATIENT TO HEAL HIMSELF.**
  At times, the patient just has no will to get well. Patient just thinks that his ailment is not curable and that he will stay sick for ever. He also thinks that no one can help him. This makes the patient keep on pulling back ill health even in spite of repeated healing done by many healers over a long period of time. In such cases; Master uses counselling as well as mental method of healing to create this desire in a patient and give him mental strength to get well.

- **A MASTER HAS DETACHED ATTACHMENT WITH PATIENT.**
  As a master has detached attachment, he just works to prepare a patient to deserve the healing. He does not expect anything. He knows that once a patient deserves good health, he is going to get it without any difficulty. This means, though he monitors the healing, he does not have any anxiety about the healing speed of a patient.

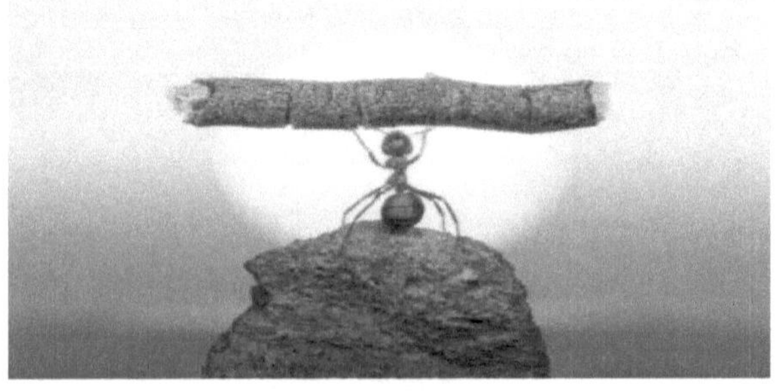

A MASTER MUST NOT USE INTENTIONS IRRESPONSIBLY.
If a master intends things without thinking properly, and gives Reiki to these intentions, even if the intention is not appropriate, still, the intentions may come true. Then the master may repent. A master must remember that unlike in Reiki 2, where Reiki takes care of your intentions and manifests ONLY things that are good for you, when a Reiki master intends anything, Reiki just supports the desire of a master and follows it unconditionally.

A MASTER MUST AVOID LOSING TEMPER.
If a master loses his temper, he may say things which may harm someone, and with his power, those things may come true. Afterwards, he may repent. So, he must be very careful now.

A MASTER MUST AVOID IRRESPONSIBLE COMMENTS AND JUDGEMENTS. HE MUST KNOW THAT HE HAS TO BE A WITNESS AND NOT A JUDGE.
A master must remember that he is just a witness. He must not judge things. On judging, if he passes some irresponsible comments, they may be improper to his image as a master and at the same time, they may also prove to be harmful to him or others at times.

A MASTER MUST AVOID EMOTIONAL INVOLVEMENT WITH PATIENT. HIS ATTACHMENT MAY DELAY THE HEALING PROCESS OF THE PATIENT.
If a master is emotionally attached with the patient, he may also have fear of failure at the back of his mind. This may come in the way of the healing of the patient and healing may get delayed.

A MASTER MUST AVOID MAKING NEGATIVE STATEMENTS THAT ARE ASSERTIVE AS HIS POWER MAY MAKE THEM TRUE AND THEN HE MAY REPENT.
If a master passes any negative assertive comments or makes any negative assertive statement, his power may bring them into reality. If he feels later that he did a mistake, may be he will not be in a position to create a contrary event by that time. So he has to be careful about saying things.

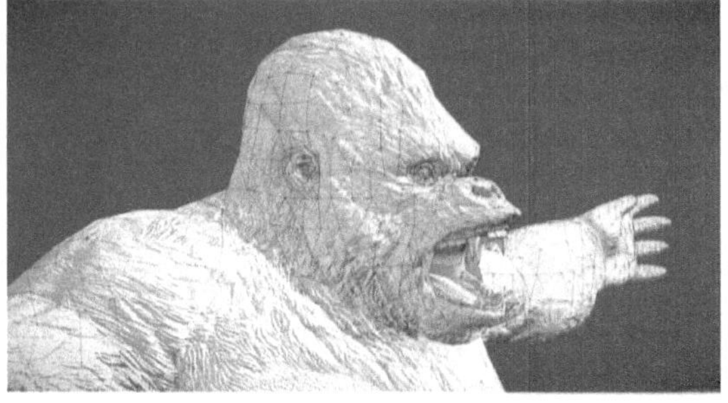

POSTURE, ATTITUDE & VOCABULARY EXPECTED OF A MASTER:

A master must be careful in using words as using wrong vocabulary may give wrong signals to the patients and others with whom a master is speaks.

At no point of time must a master indicate that he has some supernatural powers.

Master must never indicate that others are poor in awareness as compared to him.

Master must be humble in attitude and expression.

Master must live the Reiki principles in real sense and must never express any kind of anxiety or aggression or anger.

Master must never indicate any disrespect to any one in any way whatsoever.

At times, behaviour of someone deserves to invite disrespect or contempt. Yet, master must be respectful to such people.

Master must be a living expression of gratitude and service.

This certainly does not mean that a master must keep doing charity at the cost of his own living.

If a master finds people around him expecting such a charity out of him, he must politely explain that charity is something that is to be done to those who really deserve charity. Others must pay for the services of healing received out of master.

Reiki is not a matter of faith. So master must never indicate that people who wish to be treated with Reiki need to believe in it.

Master must always have a scientific, clear, respectful, polite, professional attitude where he gives respect and also maintains his own respect and space.

Even while scanning, master must never intrude the personal space of others as it is known as spiritual trace pass and though not taken as a crime on civil or criminal way, it is certainly a crime on spiritual plane. So, a master must refrain from intrusion in the personal area of a patient.

If a master finds something personal about someone while scanning, he must never discuss it with patient in public. He may request to talk to patient in privacy and then disclose his findings to the patient. This helps the patient maintain his personal space.

Even when a master finds something conclusively negative about the condition of thought formations or of the past of patient, Master must never indicate that he has seen it so clearly. Instead, he must politely ask the patient and let him talk of those negative memories.

By his soothing words, powerful posture and positively polite attitude, a master must always command respect of people around.

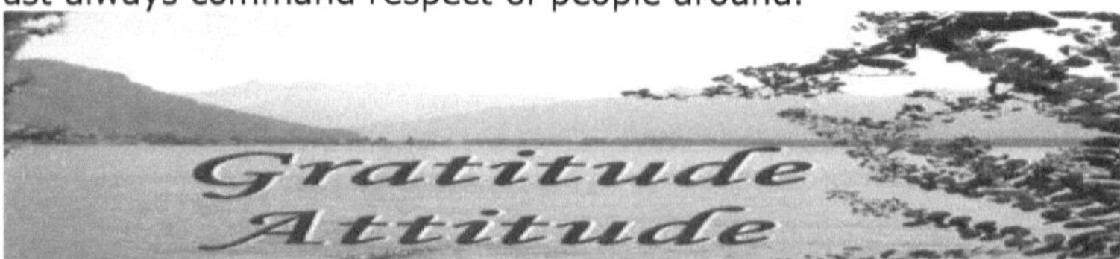

MEDITATIONS NEEDED FOR A REIKI MASTER:

A Reiki master is the one who develops all the above qualities in him slowly as he starts practicing Reiki regularly and follows the do's and don'ts of a Reiki master as given above. In addition, ideally Reiki master must regularly do some simple meditations.

Here are meditations recommended for Reiki master:

GASSHO MEDITATION

- Sit in a position that makes you feel comfortable.
- Keep your spine straight.
- Bring your hands together in prayer position but raise them above heart level, so that your index fingers are just below your chin. Let the elbows be spread so that angle of wrists is greater.
- The aim of this position is so that when you breathe out through your nose you can feel your breath on the tips of middle fingers. Adjust your hands until this is the case.
- Close your eyes.
- Focus on your breathing, check if it is fast or slow, deep or shallow. This is just because you are to be aware of it and feel the sensation of your breath on the tips of your fingers.
- Maintain the awareness of this sensation for as long as you wish. 5 to 10 minutes is good to start with, and as you get used to the practice you can lengthen the time up to half an hour or so.
- As with all meditation, and especially for beginners, you will find your mind wandering away. This can happen a lot sometimes but try not to get frustrated by this. It is natural. Your mind has probably not relaxed and focused in this manner before and it takes a while to learn that doing very little is perfectly okay.
- When you become aware of the mind wandering, just bring your attention back to your finger tips.
- Know one thing very clearly that the shopping list is allowed to wait, and that comment you made to your sister is probably long forgotten. You and your mind need attention now, the rest of the world can hang on for a bit longer.
- Once you are done this for some time, come back to the world by gently taking three long, slow and deep breaths to finish off, but that is your choice.
- Once you are finished with the meditation, take a few minutes to enjoy the peace that has taken over you and the tranquility that is now flowing through the rest of your body.
- Open your eyes, get up and start your routine.

BUDDHIST MEDITATION ON BREATHING
(ANAPANA SATI)

- Sit comfortably with hands in your lap, palms facing upwards. (As you will see later, once you have some experience, this is not necessary)
- Close your eyes.
- Become aware of your breath as in the Gassho Meditation. Is it long or slow, deep or shallow?
- Feel each in breath and feel each out breath. Some people like to mentally note "I breathe in" and "I breathe out" or to count 1 for the in breath and 2 for the out breath. Whichever method you use to maintain awareness of the breathing process, use it.
- These meditations are not trials of endurance but methods used that suit certain types of people for the reduction in stress and the production of peace.
- In this meditation, it is the awareness that matters, not the method you use to achieve it.
- Eventually, with some practice, you will realize that you are becoming much more aware of you innate self and more aware of your body as a vehicle for that self.
- This meditation can start off with 5-10 minutes and move up to 30 minutes as you progress.
- This meditation requires no special posture. So, it can be done anywhere, any time even with eyes open while you work.
- It can even make you feel a packed train as a peaceful place.
- Keep doing this as long as you wish and develop the awareness of the inner self as clearly as you can.
- Once you feel you are done, or when you feel you must get up, open your eyes. Feel the peace for some time.
- Then slowly get up and start your routine.

WATCHING THOUGHTS

- Lie down on your back.
- Place one hand on your heart & other on your naval.
- Keep looking at the roof or wall in front of you.
- Keep watching the thoughts in your mind.
- Do not resist these thoughts & do not get carried away as well.
- When your eyes become heavy, close them.
- Keep watching your thoughts even with eyes closed.
- Do this as long as you can.
- When you feel you are done, slowly open your eyes.
- Feel the inner peace that has developed in the process.
- Get up & start your routine.

REIKI PREPARATION EXERCISE
(As taught by Dr. Usui to his students)

HATSU REI HO
With thanks to Taggart King of Reiki Evolution (_http://www.reiki-evolution.co.uk_

The Reiki attunements give everyone baseline ability, so you all start off on the same footing. However, how effective or how 'clear' a channel you are depends on what you do with the energy.

It is very important to get regular practice, particularly in first few weeks after being attuned, by doing self-treatments and treating others, but from Japan has come a series of energy exercises specially designed to be used by Reiki people.

These exercises are called 'Hatsu Rei Ho'. 'Hatsu Rei Ho' originates in Tendai Buddhism, and the exercises have correspondences with Tibetan Buddhist purification rituals, Taoist or meridian massage, and QiGong too.

They are used within the Usui Reiki Ryoho Gakkai, and it was only in 1999 that the techniques were revealed in the Western world by Hiroshi Doi who is a member of Usui's Association.

Hatsu Rei Ho is designed to be carried out every day for at about 10-15 minutes, and is the basis of the practice of Reiki in the Gakkai. It is something that is done conscientiously at all First, Second & Master levels.

The Japanese word 'Ho' means 'technique', so you will find it attached to a number of Reiki techniques. 'Hatsu Rei' means 'start up Reiki', and 'Hatsu Rei Ho' can be taken as meaning a technique to start up and strengthen your Reiki.

This method, together with the Reiju empowerments that you received on the First Degree course, are the basic techniques of Usui's Reiki training as it is practised in Japan today.

Reiju is used for transmitting the Reiki ability to another person, and Hatsu Rei Ho is used to strengthen that connection and to purify the Reiki energy that passes through the student.

Hatsu Rei Ho is begun as soon as the student starts training with the Gakkai, and students would receive Reiju empowerments every week, to enhance their intuitive abilities and accelerate their spiritual development.

It was taught that it is not enough simply to receive a Reiki empowerment, although the Reiki ability will never leave you. If a student wanted to progress on their spiritual path, they needed to do three things:

- ξ Continue to receive Reiju empowerments on a regular basis,
- ξ Practice Hatsu Rei Ho daily,
- ξ Live the 'Reiki Principles' as part of their life.

Stage One: Relax

Relax and close your eyes, and place your hands palms down on your lap. Focus your attention on your Tanden point:
(an energy centre two fingerbreadths (3-5 cm) below your tummy button and 1/3 of the way into your body.)

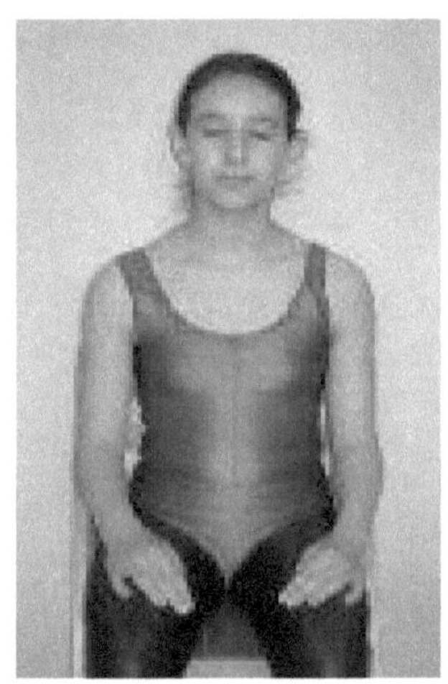

Stage Two: Mokunen (Focusing)

Say to yourself "I'm going to start Hatsu Rei now".

Stage Three: Kenyoku

This means 'Dry Bathing' or 'Brushing Off'

Kenyoku can be seen as a way of getting rid of negative energy. It has correspondences with Taoist massage, or meridian massage.

Here is what to do:

Place the fingertips of your right hand near the top of the left shoulder, where the collarbone meets bulge of shoulder.

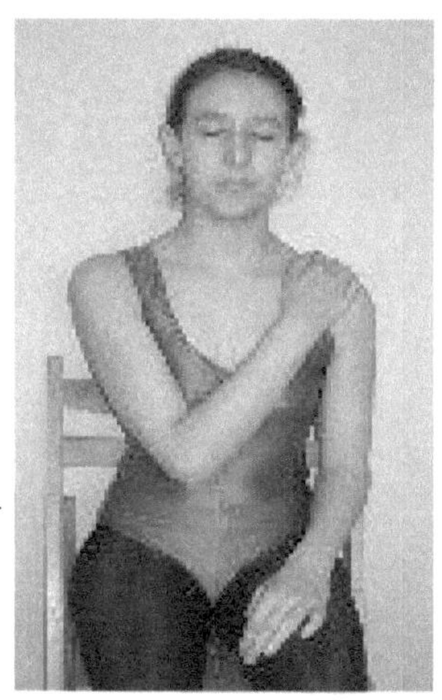

The hand is lying flat on chest.

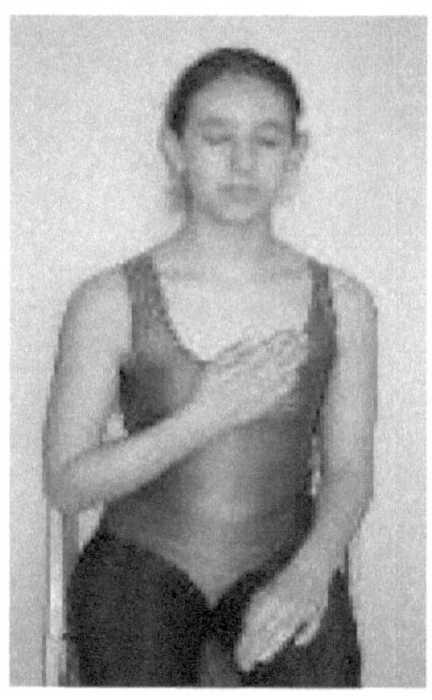

Draw your flat hand down and across the chest in a straight line, over the base of the sternum *(where your breastbone stops and your abdomen starts, in the midline)*

Draw your flat hand further down to the right hip.

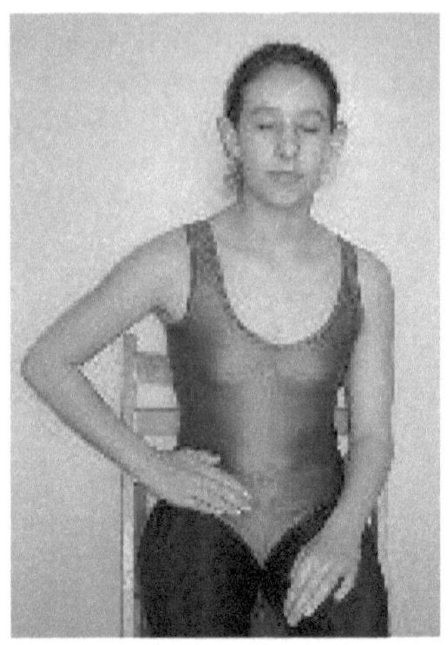

Exhale as you do this.

Place the fingertips of your left hand near the top of the right shoulder, where the collarbone meets bulge of shoulder.

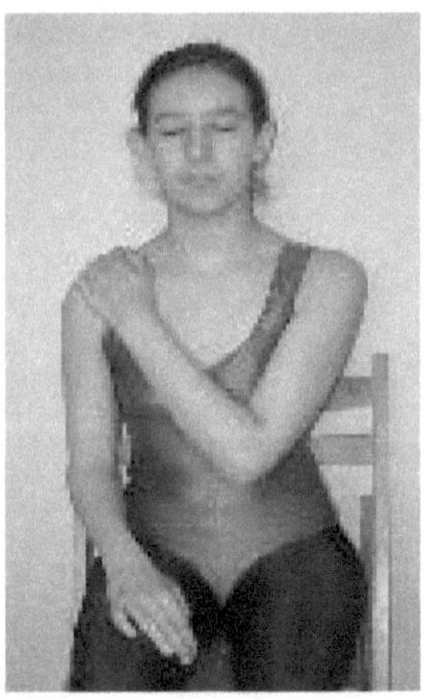

The hand is lying flat on your chest.

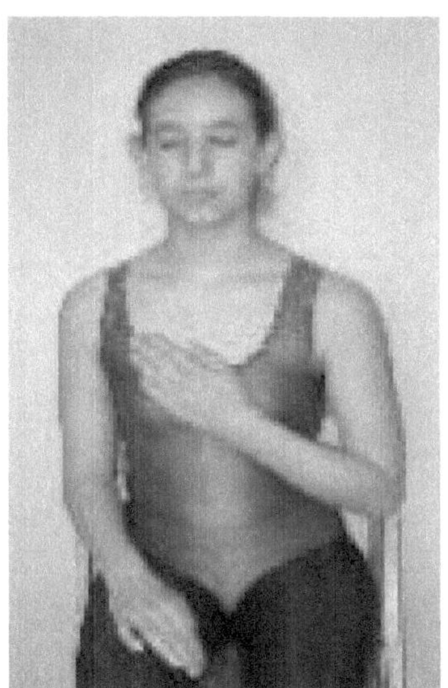

Draw your flat hand down and across the chest in a straight line, over the base of the sternum *(where your breastbone stops and your abdomen starts, in the midline)*

Draw your flat hand further down to the right hip.

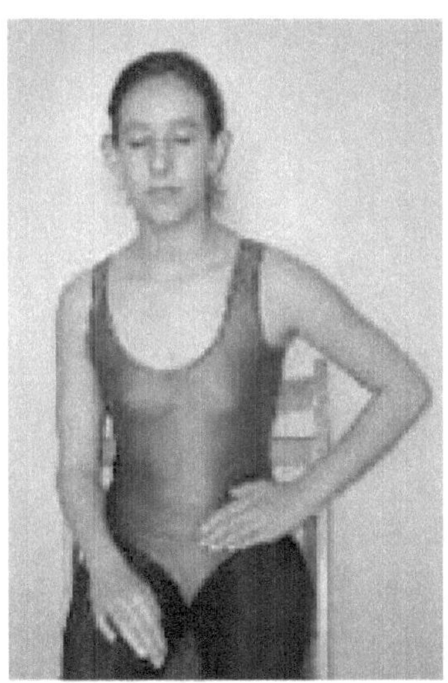

Exhale as you do this.

Inhale and again, draw your right hand from left shoulder, in a straight line across the sternum, to the right hip, and again exhale as you make the downward movement.

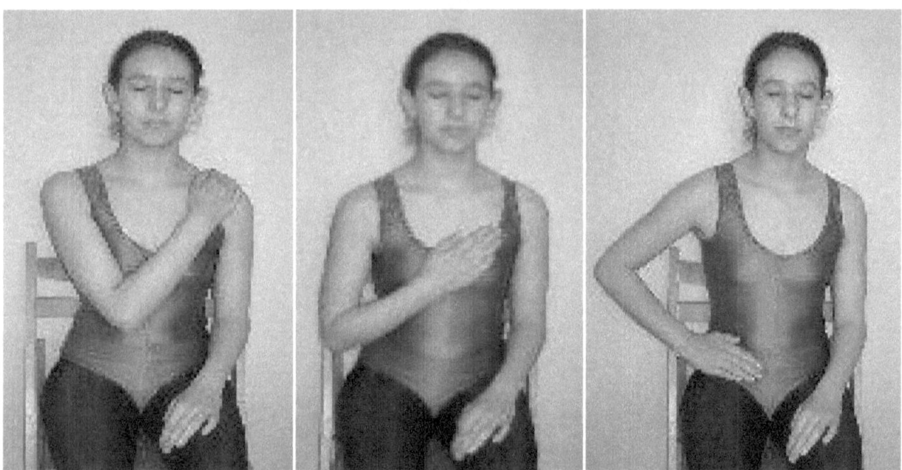

Inhale and again draw your left hand from the right shoulder, in a straight line across the sternum, to the left hip, and again exhale as you make the downward movement.

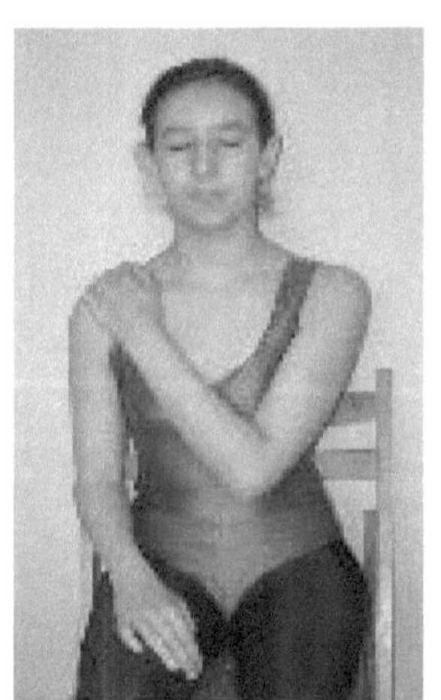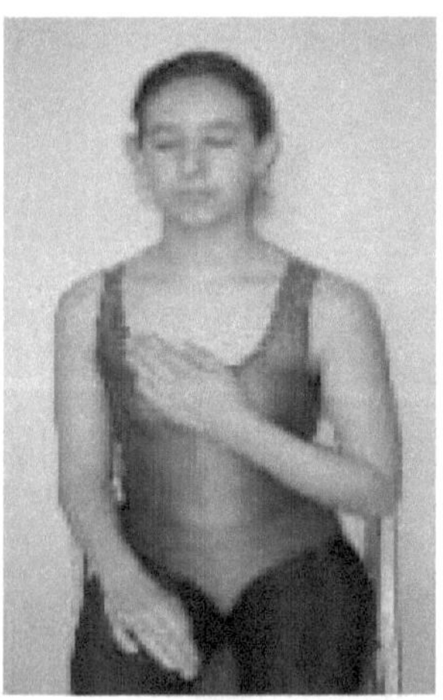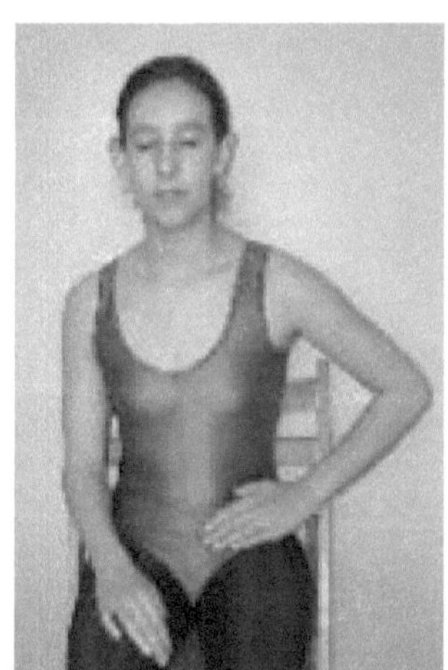

Inhale and again, draw your right hand from left shoulder, in a straight line across the sternum, to the right hip, and again exhale as you make the downward movement.

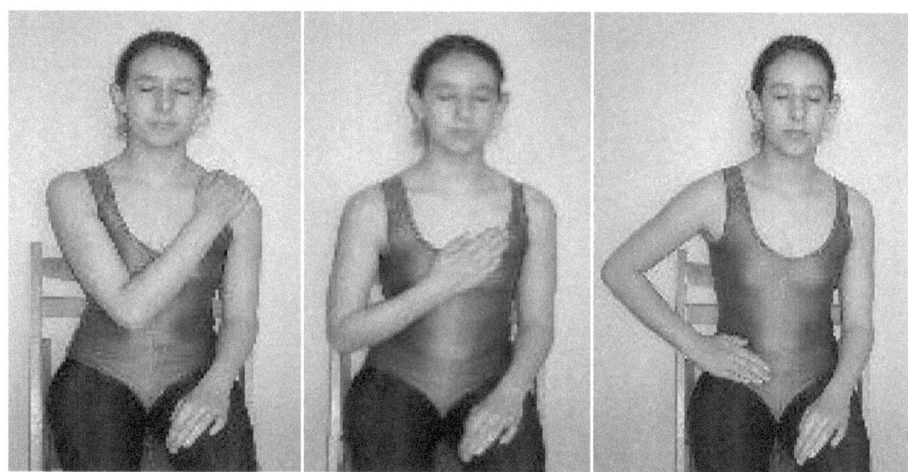

Inhale and again draw your left hand from the right shoulder, in a straight line across the sternum, to the left hip, and again exhale as you make the downward movement.

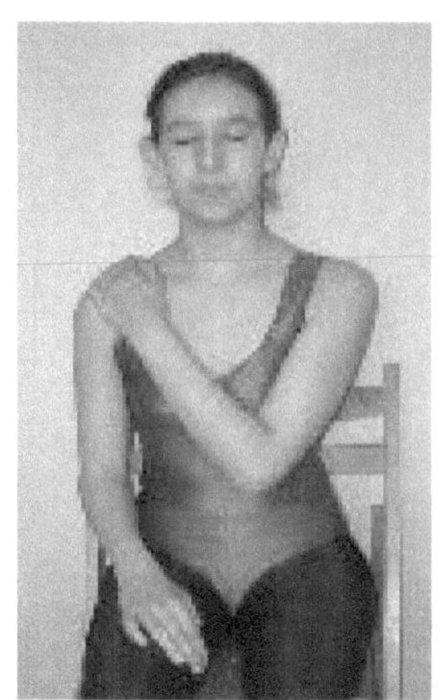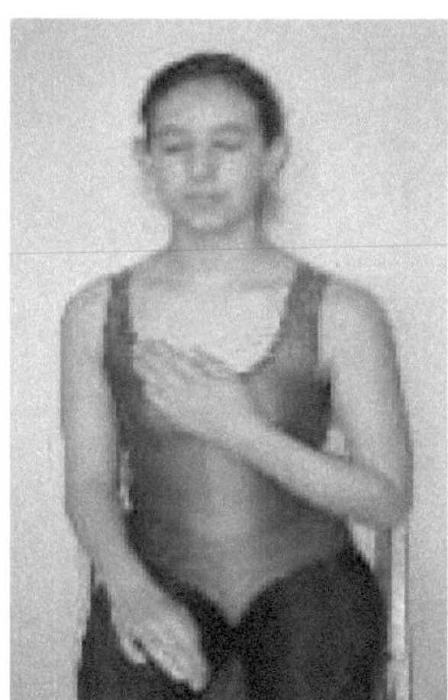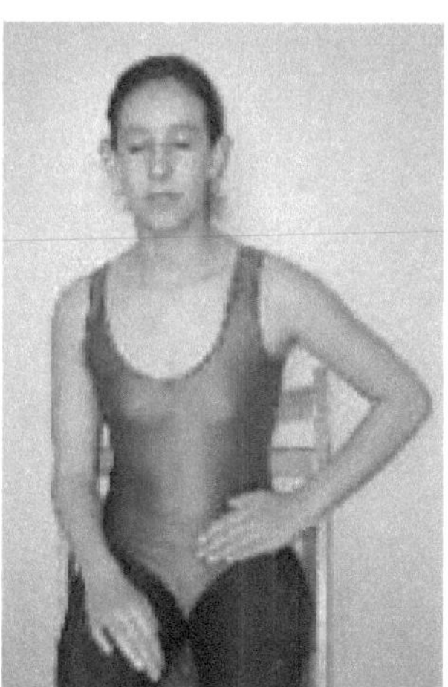

Inhale. Now put your right fingertips on the outer edge of the left shoulder, at the top of your slightly outstretched left arm, with your fingertips pointing sideways away from your body.

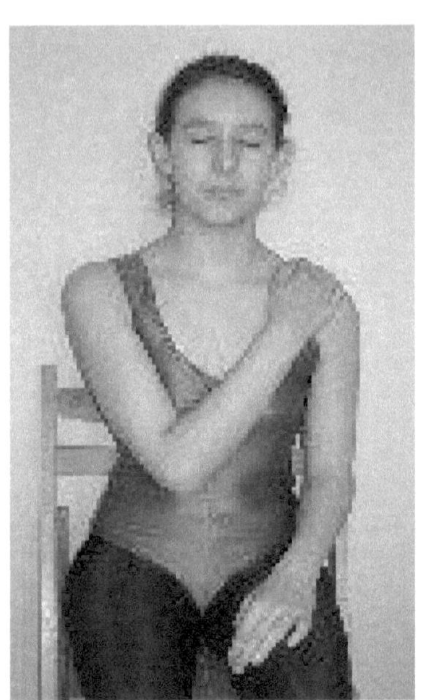

Move your right hand, flattened, along the outside of your arm.

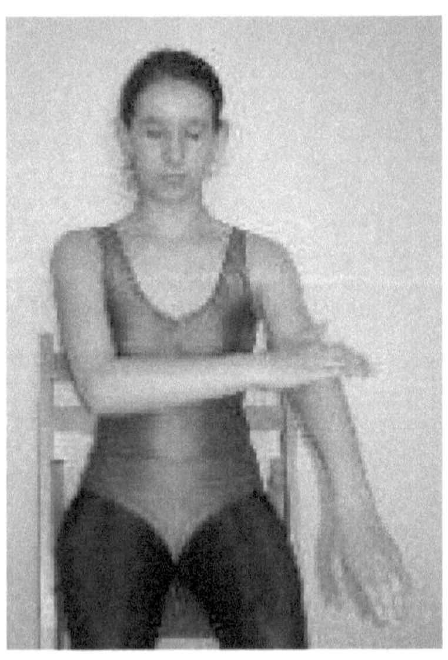

Keep, your hand moving all the way to the fingertips and beyond, all the while keeping the left arm straight. Exhale as you do this.

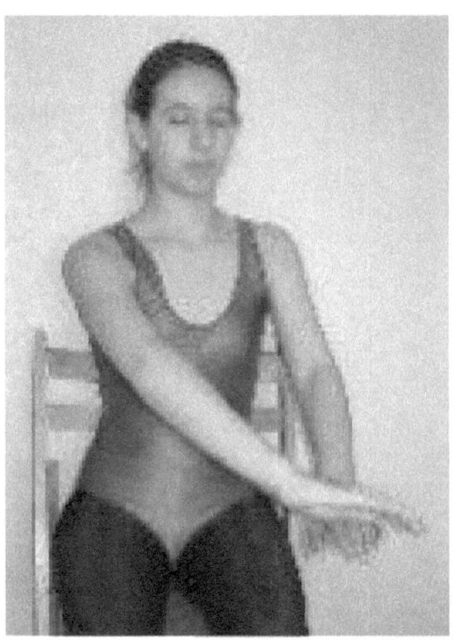

Inhale. Now put your left fingertips on the outer edge of the right shoulder, at the top of your slightly outstretched right arm, with your fingertips pointing sideways away from your body.

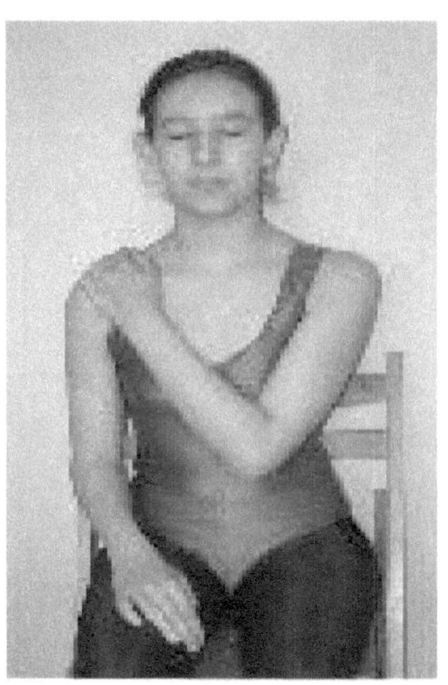

Move your left hand, flattened, along the outside of your right arm,

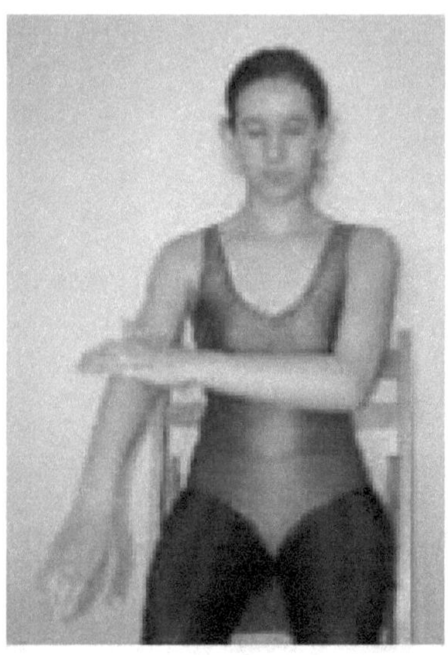

Keep the hand moving all the way to the fingertips and beyond, all the while keeping the right arm straight. Exhale as you do this.

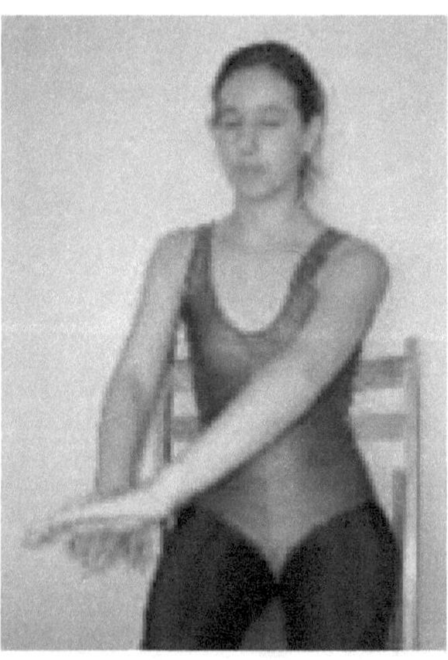

Inhale. Repeat the process on left side with right fingertips again, Exhale as you do this.

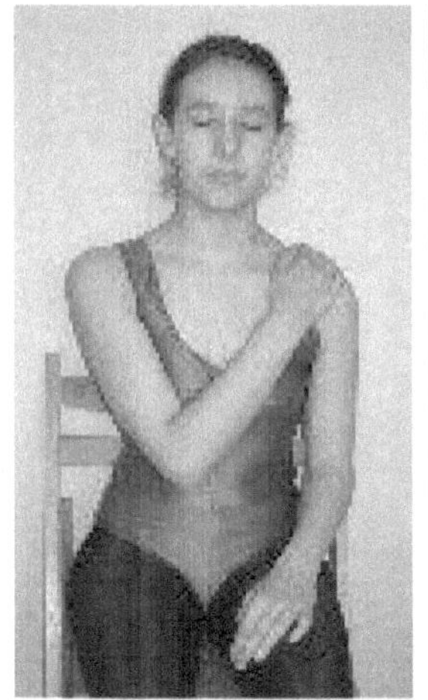 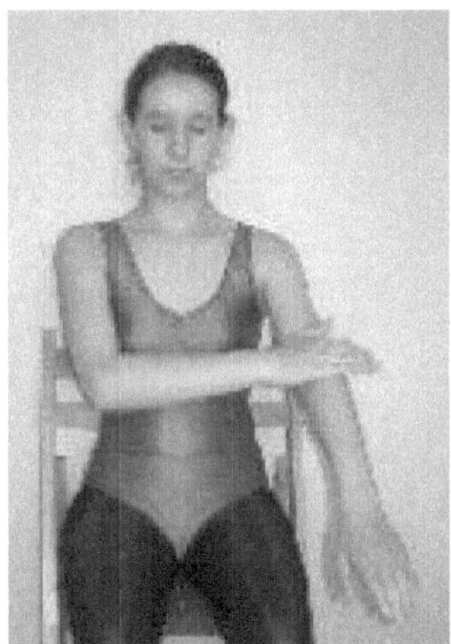 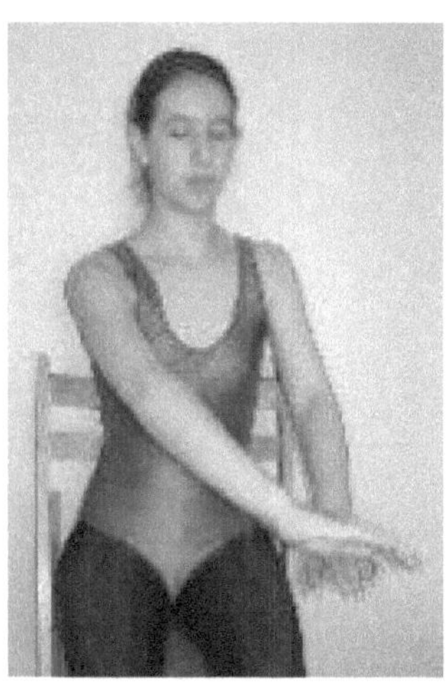

Inhale. Repeat the process on right side with left fingertips again, Exhale as you do this.

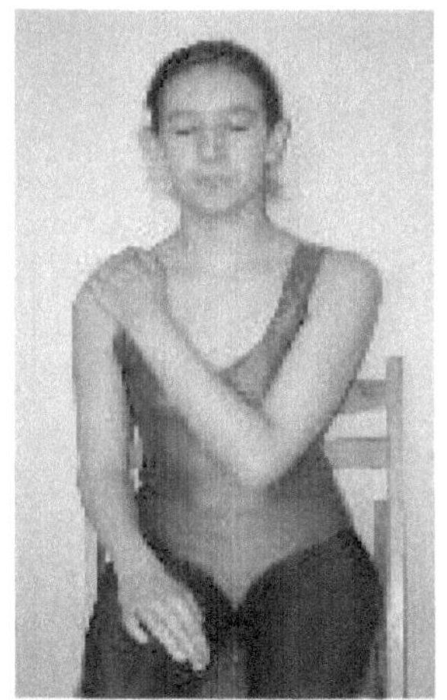 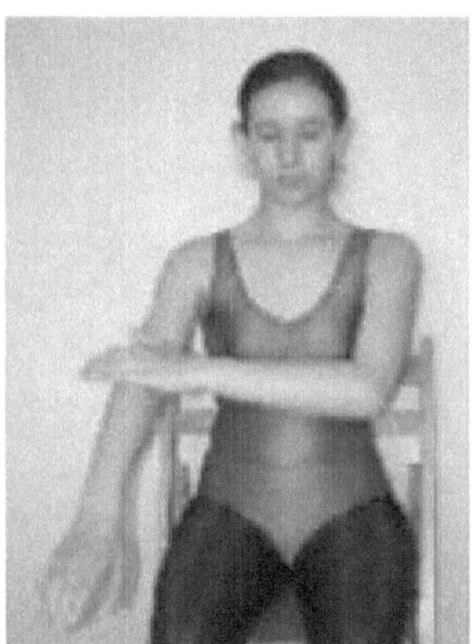 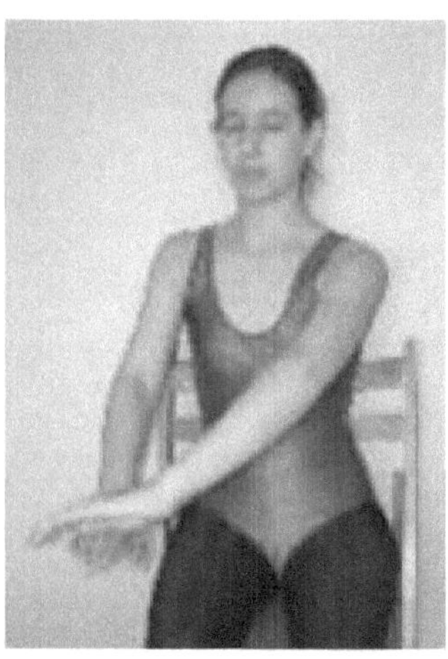

Inhale. Repeat the process on left side with right fingertips again, Exhale as you do this.

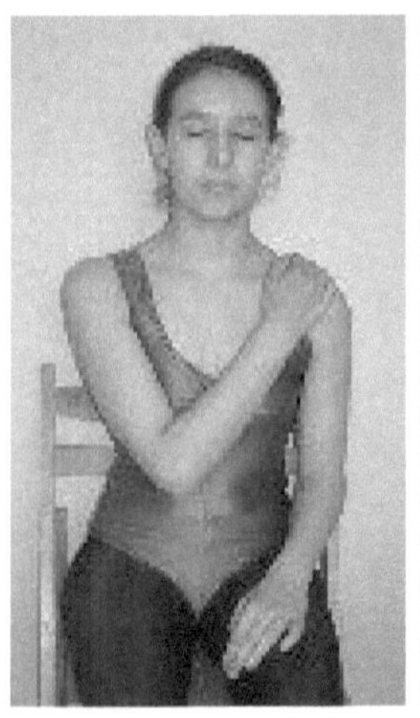 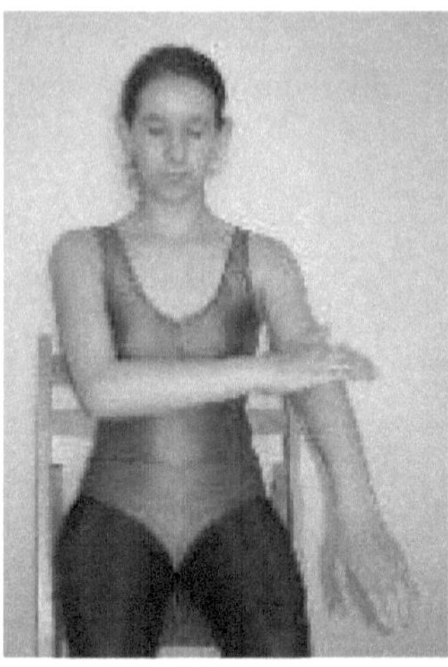 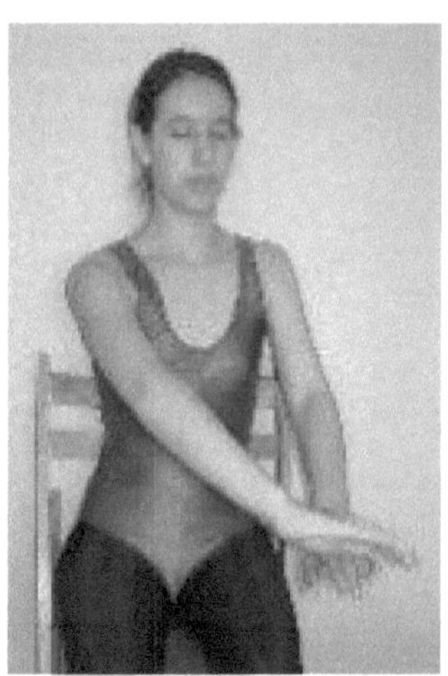

Inhale. Repeat the process on right side with left fingertips again, Exhale as you do this.

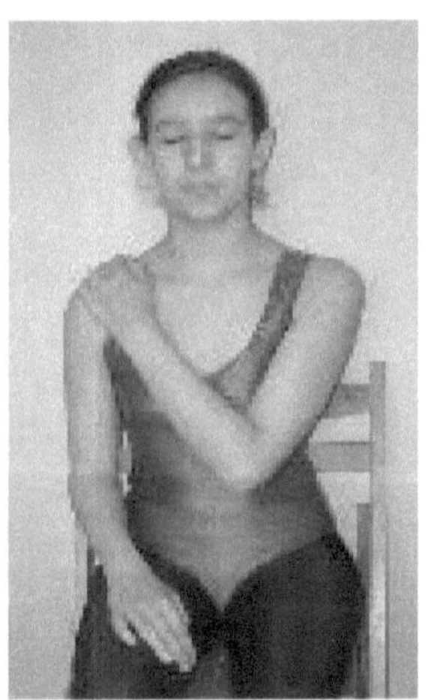 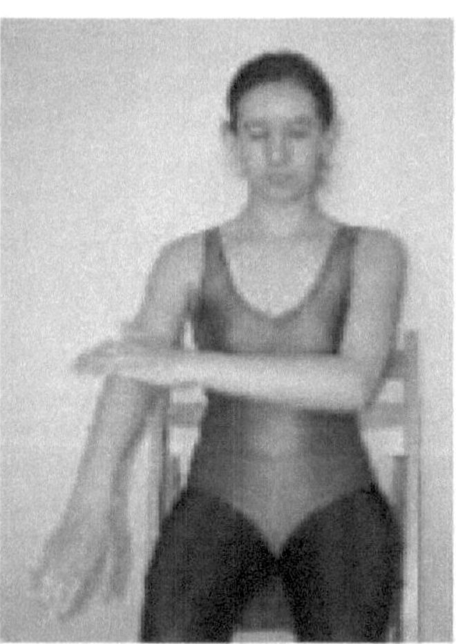 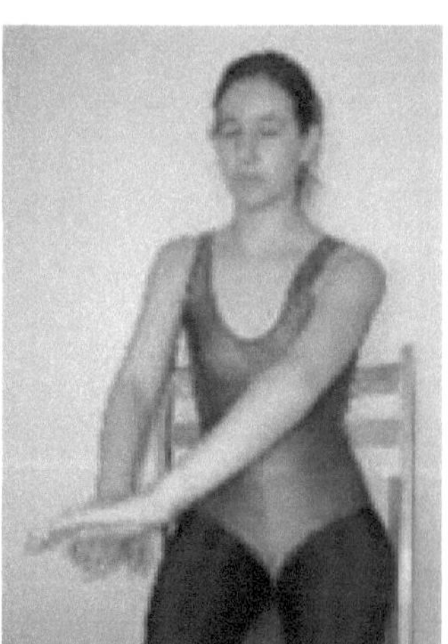

Stage Four: Connect to Reiki

Raise your hands high up in air on either side of head, with palms facing sky & fingers pointing towards midline.
Visualize energy / white light entering your hands running through your arms into body & connect to Reiki.

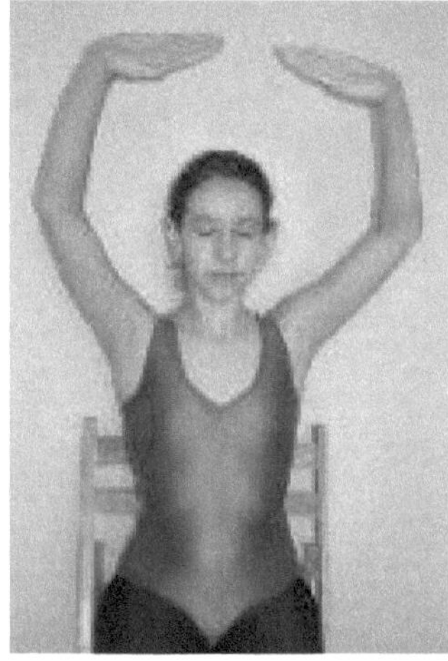

Feel the sensations as you become aware of Reiki flowing, slowly lower your hands.
This position is the first of the "Eight Brocades" in Qi Gong: connecting heaven and earth.

Stage Five: Joshin Kokkyu Ho

This means "Technique for Purification of the Spirit" or "Soul Cleansing Breathing Method".
This is a meditation that focuses on the Tanden point.

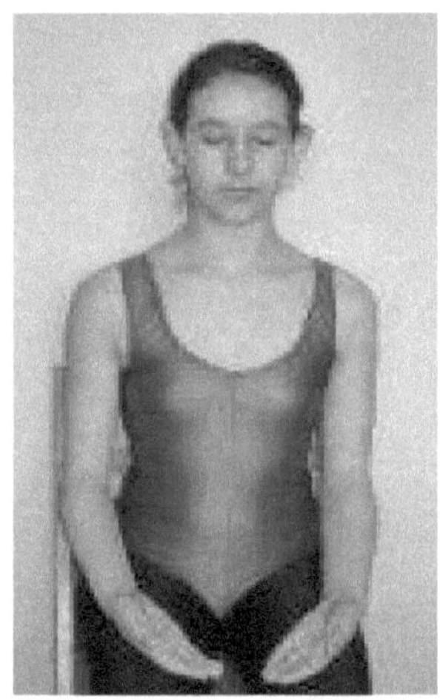

Put your hands on your lap with your palms facing upwards and breathe naturally through your nose.

Focus on your Tan den point and relax.

When you breathe in, visualize energy or light flooding into your crown chakra and passing into your Tan den and, as you pause before exhaling, feel that energy expand throughout your body, melting all your tensions.

Feel energy / tingling in your hands and feet, as meditation progresses.

Stay with this energy for some time.

Stage Six: Gassho

Gassho means "hands together", and the correct position to hold is to have your hands together in front of your chest (like praying hands) a little higher that your heart, so that you could breathe out onto your fingertips.

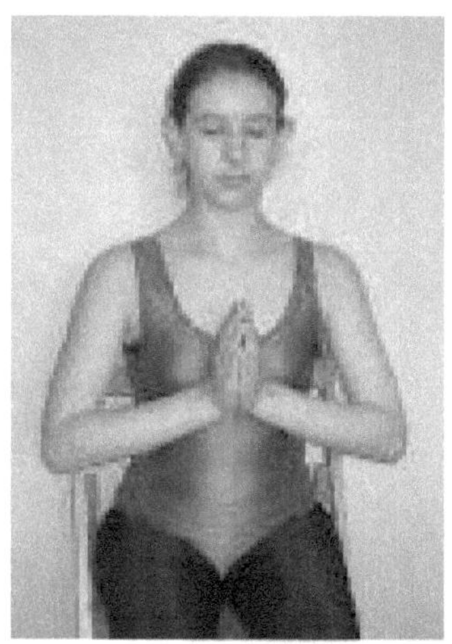

Hold this position for meditation.

An important aspect of this meditation is that you should focus your awareness on the point where your middle fingers touch.

You might try putting your tongue up to touch the roof of your mouth with each in-breath, and release the tongue on each out-breath, and see if this makes any difference to your experience of this stage.

Stage Seven: Seishin Toitsu

This means "my mind is focused" or "my spirit is gathered", and is the stage when Reiju is given by teachers in the Gakkai.

Stay in the Gassho position.

When you breathe in, visualize energy or light flooding into your hands & passing into your Tan den: breathe in through your hands.

Feel the energy accumulating there.

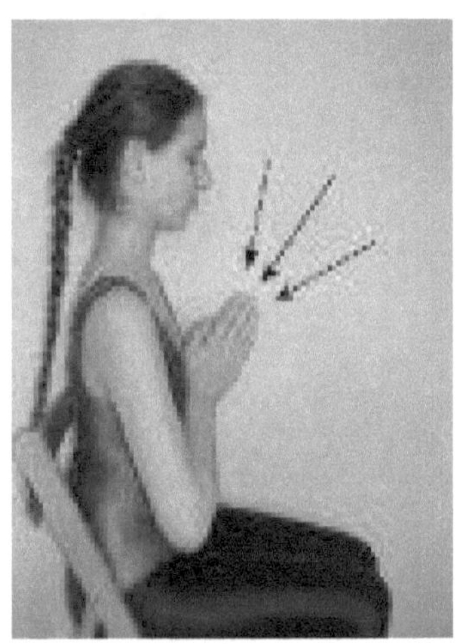

When you breathe out, visualize that the energy stored in your tan den floods out through your hands.

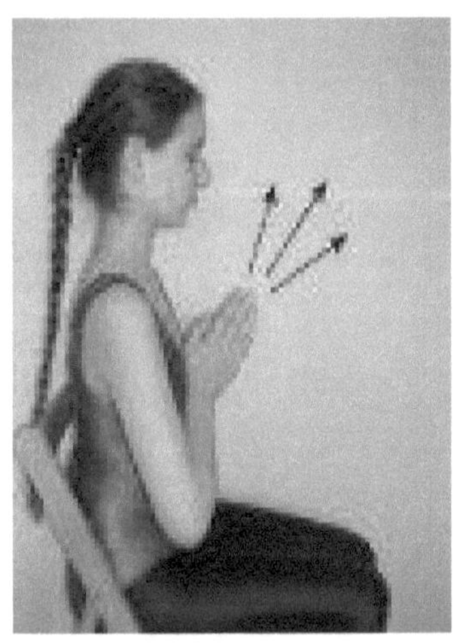

Stage Eight: Gokai Sansho

Say the 5 Principles aloud, three times.
- **JUST FOR TODAY, I WILL NOT GET ANGERY.**
- **JUST FOR TODAY, I WILL NOT BE WORRIED.**
- **JUST FOR TODAY, I WILL BE HONEST IN LIFE.**
- **JUST FOR TODAY, I WILL LOVE & RESPECT ALL.**
- **JUST FOR TODAY, I WILL BE THANKFUL TO ALL.**

Stage Nine: Mokunen

Put your hands back on to your laps with your palms down. Say "I've finished Hatsu Rei Ho now" to your sub-conscious.

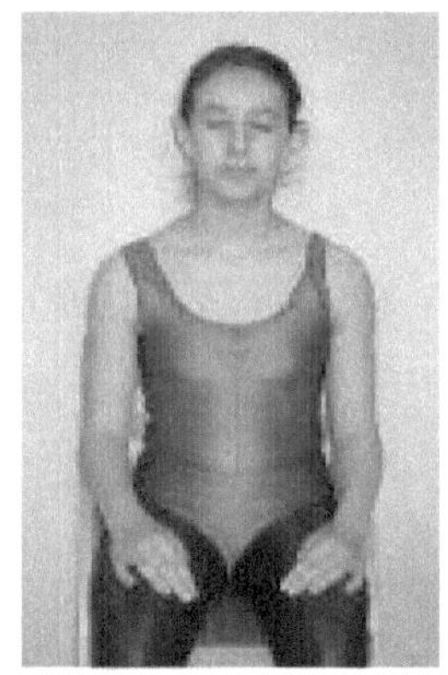

Open your eyes and shake your hands up/down/left/right for a few seconds.

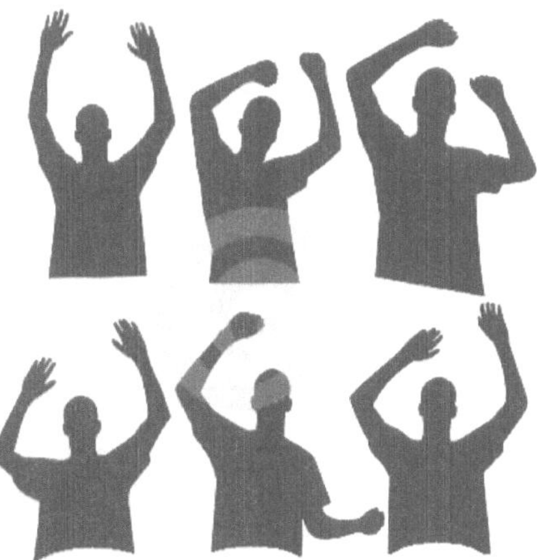

Start your routine.

ANOTHER WAY of HATSUREI-HO:

Hatsurei-Ho:

1. ***Preparation*** – clear the mind with introspection by sitting quiet for 2 minutes.

   Use Gyosei.

   Chant "Om Mani Padme Hum" for 2 minutes.

2. ***Kihon Shisei*** - sit in zazen style.

   To sit in zazen, bend your legs and place the left knee on the floor.

   Place the right knee down about two fist widths from the left.

   Now flip down the toes and place the feet onto the floor so that the big toes just touch each other.

   Lower the buttocks down so that they rest on or between the heels.

   Straighten up and let the lower back move forward so that there is an S shaped curve to the spine.

   Rounding out the lower back to the rear or trying to sit back too far will cause muscle fatigue.

   The weight should be centred somewhere between the top of the feet and the knees, more toward the feet.

   The head is carried in balance on top of the spine.

   The ears should be in line with the shoulders and the nose in line with the belly button.

   Note that putting the nose into this position moves the back ever so slightly off of a strictly vertical position.

   In Iai this is important, as it will encourage "seme" or pressure to the front.

   Pull the chin in slightly and stretch the back of the neck.

   This should feel as if someone is pulling straight up on the hair to stretch the spine.

   To find this centreline you can rock in circles from the hips, slowly reducing the swings until coming to rest in a stable position.

This centring is important to prevent muscle cramps or fatigue while sitting.

Another way to check the posture is to imagine a string attached to the top of the head on the inside.

The string drops down inside the neck and trunk and is attached to a weight at the height of your tanden.

If you bend your head forward or curve your trunk too much the string touches the body shell.

If you lean too far forward or back the weight bangs into the hip girdle.
Put the weight in the front half of the hara.

Relax the shoulders and let the arms fall downward naturally.

The right hand is placed palm upward on the lap with the little finger edge lightly touching the lower abdomen.

The left hand is placed on top of the right, palm upward as well.

The fingers should be together without strain.

Place the tips of the thumbs together so that they are just touching with no pressure.

The thumbs and fingers should make an oval shape around a point about 2 to 3 inches below the navel.

[This point is called the tanden or seika tanden and corresponds roughly to the centre of balance. The left hand over the right represents the calm ("Sei" or "In" in Japanese) aspects covering the active ("Do" or "Yo") aspects. The thumbs unify the two. The tanden is seen as the centre of being around which the Hara or hip girdle is organized. The centre is the point from which your life is lived. Variations of this form are sometimes used but this is the most balanced and relaxed method of sitting.]

3. **Mokunen** – set the intent of your focus with a clear mind and with mindfulness say, "I am beginning Hatsurei now" to both the mind and the subconscious.

4. **Kenyoku-Ho** – place your right hand, fingertips facing up, on your left shoulder.

The fingertips should be touching the shoulder and the palm flat on chest.

Slide your hand downwards toward your right hip (your hand must remain in contact with your body) until your fingertips are at your right hip.

Repeat for the opposite side, using your left hand.

Once finished, place your right hand in left armpit and slide hand down to left fingertips.

Repeat for the opposite side, using your left hand.

Once finished, place your right hand, palm down, on top of your left forearm (at elbow) and slide hand down to left fingertips.

Repeat for the opposite side, using your left hand.

5. ***Jyoshin Koki-Ho*** – place your hands in Gassho, eyes closed, and breathing in through the nose and out through the mouth.

When you breathe in through the nose, visualise a white mist or light entering your nose, going into the crown and ending up in your Hara.

When you breathe out through the mouth, visualise the white mist or light going out into the universe, but with the white light still remaining in the Hara.

6. ***Gassho*** – hands are clasped together in prayer position in front of the chest; middle fingers are straight with fingertips touching. Some people call this the "Reiki Laser".

Say the Reiki Principles: "For today only, anger not, worry not, be humble, work with gratitude on yourself, and be kind to all".

Say three times.

7. ***Mokunen*** – set the intent of your focus with a clear mind and with mindfulness say, "I am finished with Hatsurei now" to both the mind and the subconscious.

8. **Hatsurei-Ho** is now finished.

5 PILLARS OF REIKI MASTER'S HEALING:

Healing of a Traditional Reiki master is based on the following 4 pillars:

First Pillar of Reiki practice: Reiki Principles

A Reiki master not only remembers, but also lives all 5 Reiki principles. These Reiki principles are actually the **Five Reiki Precepts** (五戒 *Gokai*, meaning "The Five Commandments", from the Buddhist teachings against killing, thievery, sexual misconduct, lying, and intemperance) **taught by Dr. Usui as a foundation of his** Reiki teachings.

These traditionally taught Reiki principles are as follows:

6. JUST FOR TODAY, I WILL NOT GET ANGERY.
7. JUST FOR TODAY, I WILL NOT BE WORRIED.
8. JUST FOR TODAY, I WILL BE HONEST IN LIFE.
9. JUST FOR TODAY, I WILL LOVE & RESPECT ALL.
10. JUST FOR TODAY, I WILL BE THANKFUL TO ALL.

A Reiki master makes them a part of his being in leading normal life.

Second pillar of Reiki practice: Effective Breathing

Though the specific use of breath and breathing is central to many styles of Japanese Reiki, it is often a neglected topic in Western Reiki.

Usui taught a technique called ***Joshin Kokyū-hō*** (女神呼吸法), which roughly translates as "the breathing method for cleansing the spirit," though literally translates as "Goddess Breath Method".

Joshin Kokyū-hō is performed by sitting straight, with the back aligned, breathing in slowly through the nose.

As the practitioner inhales, s/he also breathes the Reiki energy in through the crown Chakra in order to purify the body and make it fit for the flow of Reiki, and is drawn down into the tanden.

Tanden is the energy centre located deep inside a chakra that stores energy. *The word **Tanden** is the Japanese equivalent of the Chinese: **Tan Tien** (also: dan tian) or field of the elixir.*

There are three main tandens in body; they are in following positions:

1: Deep inside Hara;
[The Lower (*Shimo*) Tanden (also: *Ge Tanden or Seika tandon*)]
2: Inside the chest at about heart level;
[The Middle (*Naka*) Tanden (also: *Chu Tanden*)
3: Inside Third eye;
[The Upper (*Kami*) Tanden (also: *Jo Tanden*)

Seika tanden is taken to be the main tanden of these three. This is why it is commonly referred to simply as the *tanden.*

The term *Seika* simply refers to 'below the Navel'. The *Seika tanden* is an energy 'centre' or area - about the size of a grapefruit - located deep inside Hara, roughly mid way between the top of the pubic bone and the navel. *Seika Tanden* is also known as *the Kikai* ('Ocean of Ki') *Tanden*, and as *Seika no Itten* (the 'One Point' below the Navel). In some western Energy Disciplines this point is referred to as the 'Lunar Plexus'.

Physically speaking it is the body's center of gravity. It is said that Ki is moved by the mind that is why, we say, where the attention goes, ki flows. To effortlessly focus the *awareness* (thought-feeling) in *seika tanden* is to place one's energy there. Also, by placing effortless emphasis and energy at this area in the lower abdomen, integration of body and mind is deepened and strengthened, and the Spirit is dynamically grounded in the Present Moment. This is certainly not the same as *concentration or willfulness.*

Traditional Japanese disciplines - martial, spiritual, therapeutic or artistic - tend to speak of a *single* tanden. However, in Japan there are several disciplines - either of Chinese origin or alternatively heavily influenced by Chinese Chi Gung philosophy.

Many of these disciplines speak of *three* tandens:

The Lower (*Shimo*) Tanden (also: *Ge Tanden*) [essentially the same as the *seika tanden*] - located deep inside the 'hara'

The Middle (*Naka*) Tanden (also: *Chu Tanden*) - located inside the chest at about the heart level

The Upper (*Kami*) Tanden (also: *Jo Tanden*) - located in the middle of the head between the eyes

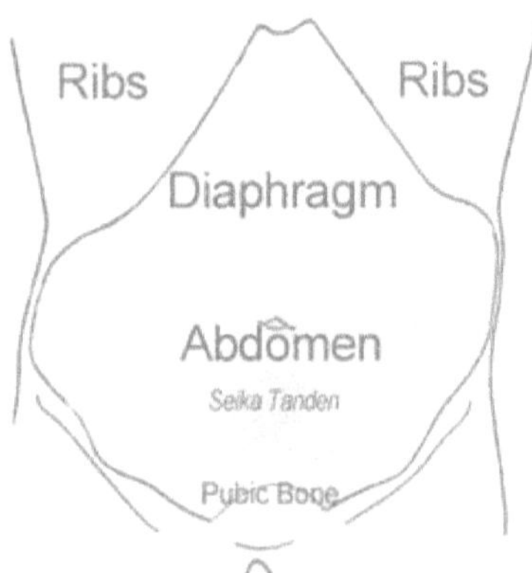

Position of Seika Tanden

Other Three pillars: Gassho, Reiji-ho & Chiryo

Along with the five Reiki principles, Usui based his Reiki system on three other practises; *Gasshō*, *Reiji-hō*, and *Chiryō*.

Gasshō

Gasshō ("合掌" in Japanese, meaning "two hands coming together") is a meditative state where both palms of the hands are placed together.

Earlier, this method was taken to be the starting point of Reiki and was practised each time at the beginning of Usui's Reiki workshops and meetings.

One technique of Gasshō is to concentrate on the pads where the two middle fingers meet. (Check for the Gasshō meditation given above)

Reiji-hō

Reiji-hō (霊示法, meaning "indication of the Reiki power method") is a means of connecting with the Reiki power by asking it to flow through the practitioner three times, and is commonly split into three parts.

The first part is to ask the Reiki power to flow through the practitioner. It will either enter through the crown chakra (as this is the highest ascension), the heart chakra (as indicated by the pure love of Reiki), or the hands (as the palms are attuned with specific Reiki symbols).

A student of the Second Degree can use the third/distance symbol to connect with the Reiki along with the first/power symbol; the distance symbol is sent first and is then sealed with the power symbol.

The second part is to pray for the recovery of the person if a specific ailment is being healed, or for the general health of the person if otherwise.

The third part is to place both hands, palms facing each other, to the third eye (the area in between the two eyebrows), and ask the Reiki power to guide the hands to where energy is needed.

Though similar to the practice of *Byosen-hō*, *Reiji-hō* relies specifically on intuition of where to heal, whereas *Byosen-hō* scans for areas with the hands, feeling for subtle changes in the aura of the practitioner's hands and the aura of the recipient.

Chiryō

Chiryō ["治療" in Japanese, meaning "(medical) treatment"] requires the practitioner to place his/her dominant hand on the crown chakra and wait for hibiki (響き, "feedback") in the form of an impulse or inspiration, which the hand then follows. During Chiryō, the practitioner gives free rein to the hand, touching painful areas of the body until the area no longer hurts or until the hands move on their own to another area

THINGS YOU CAN WORK ON WITH REIKI 3:

- SCAN & HEAL ANYONE ANYWHERE

- SCAN EVENTS & CHECK THEIR POSSIBILITY

- SPEED UP ONES OWN SPIRITUAL GROWTH

- DETECT EMOTION BEHIND PROBLEM & HEAL IT

- CREATE THE DESIRE IN PATIENT TO GET WELL

- GIVE BASIC COUNSELLING WHILE HEALING

- HEAL WITH DETACHED ATTACHMENT

- HEAL WITH COMMAND OVER NATURE & ENERGY

- CREATE +VE EVENTS OF CHOICE WITH NO LIMIT

BENEFITS OF REIKI 4 OVER REIKI 3
= WHY IS IT ADVISABLE NOT TO STOP REIKI QUEST AT REIKI 3?

- REIKI 3 HELPS US TO SCAN DISTANT THINGS AND PERSONS.
- IT OPENS THE ABILITY OF DISTANCE DIAGNOSIS IN A HEALER.
- BUT REIKI 4 TEACHES US TO USE THIS WITH ABSOLUTE ACCURACY.
- WITH REIKI 4, WE CAN DETECT THE PROBLEM & HEAL IT UPTO A SINGLE NERVE OR SINGLE CELL LEVEL.
- THIS KIND OF PRECISION IS NOT AVAILABLE EVEN IN MOST ADVANCED SURGERIES TILL DATE, BUT A REIKI 4 HEALER CAN PERFORM HEALING WITH THIS LEVEL OF ACCURACY.
- ACU-REIKI LEARNED AT REIKI 4 LEVEL HELP A HEALER TO GIVE INSTANT HEALING RESULT TO PATIENT EVEN IN SEVERE PROBLEM.
- REIKI DOWSING NOT ONLY HELPS A HEALER DO ACCURATE DIAGNOSIS, BUT ALSO HELP|S HIM TO RECORD THE HEALING AND PRESENT A RECORDED EVIDENCE OF HEALING WHICH HE CAN ALWAYS CROSS CHECK WITH REPORTS OF MEDICAL CHECK UPS.
- REIKI 4 TEACHES BASIS ANATOMY THAT IS MANDATORY FOR A HEALER BUT NEVER BTAUGHT IN ANY OTHER REIKI CLASSES.
- REIKI 4 MEDITATIONS HELP A HEALER TO STAY PROTECTED.
- ADVANCED SYMBOLS OF REIKI 4 CAN OVERCOME ALL POSSIBLE LIMITS THAT EVEN MANY REIKI MASTERS FACED IN HEALING.

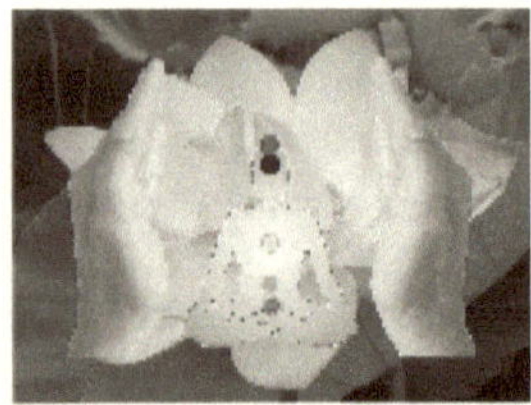

ξ   Reiki is a very simple method to heal any ailment just by touch or thought.
ξ   Anyone can learn these three levels of Reiki just with training of 3 hours per levels.
ξ   This book contains a detailed and exhaustive study material followed during the Reiki training by Intentional Healing Foundation teachers.
ξ   Even other Reiki teachers may use this study material for their Reiki classes, with the written consent of the author, with the help of this book.
ξ   Those who have learned Reiki, can use this book to refresh their study and practice Reiki with greater efficiency.

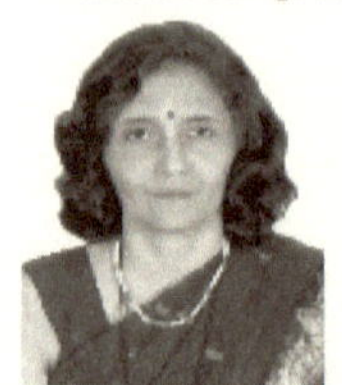

- Dr. Rekhaa kale is master in Philosophy & Psychology.
- She has been teaching Logic & Psychology since 1978.
- She is a Medical Doctor with a degree in Homeopathy.
- She is a Post Graduate in Law & Human Rights.
- She is working since 1991 in the area of healing.
- She has astral communication with spiritual masters.
- She astrally received symbols & methods from Dr. Mikao Usui
- In 1992, she developed intentional healing system.

@   Intentional Healing works to heal body by healing emotions.
@   She subscribes to medical sciences view that ailments originate in mind.
@   You can learn more about handling anger & solve problems, with author.
@   Contact author on: **rekhaa.kale@yahoo.com**, or 9820044254 / 9870044254

OTHER BOOKS BY AUTHOR:

@   **EASY GUIDE TO REIKI** — PUBLISHED BY FUSION BOOKS, DIAMOND PUBLICATION, IN 2005
@   **EASY GUIDE TO DOWSING** — PUBLISHED BY FUSION BOOKS; DIAMOND PUBLICATION, IN 2007
@   **EASY GUIDE TO FENG SHUI** — PUBLISHED BY FUSION BOOKS; DIAMOND PUBLICATION, IN 2004
@   **EASY GUIDE TO MEDITATION** — PUBLISHED BY FUSION BOOKS; DIAMOND PUBLICATION, IN 2005
@   **EASY GUIDE TO PEACE OF MIND** — PUBLISHED BY FUSION BOOKS; DIAMOND PUBLICATION, IN 2005
@   **EASY GUIDE TO RELATIONSHIP BUILDING** — PUBLISHED BY FUSION BOOKS; DIAMOND PUBLICATION, IN 2005
@   **PAST LIFE A MYSTIQUE REALITY** — PUBLISHED BY FUSION BOOKS; DIAMOND PUBLICATION, IN 2012

To get these books, contact Diamond books on: 011 41611861 / info@dpb.in / sales@dpb.in

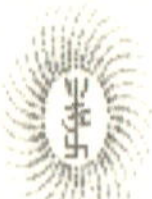

INTENTIONAL HEALING FOUNDATION

http://way2health.webs.com

intentionalhealingfoundation@yahoo.com

Rs. 797/-

www.ingramcontent.com/pod-product-compliance
Lightning Source LLC
Chambersburg PA
CBHW051056250726
48656CB00001B/331